The Healing Trail:
Essential Oils of Madagascar

Georges Halpern, M.D., Ph.D.
with Peter Weverka

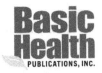
Basic
Health
PUBLICATIONS, INC.

The information contained in this book is based upon the research and personal and professional experiences of the authors. It is not intended as a substitute for consulting with your physician or other healthcare provider. Any attempt to diagnose and treat an illness should be done under the direction of a healthcare professional.

The publisher does not advocate the use of any particular healthcare protocol but believes the information in this book should be available to the public. The publisher and authors are not responsible for any adverse effects or consequences resulting from the use of the suggestions, preparations, or procedures discussed in this book. Should the reader have any questions concerning the appropriateness of any procedures or preparation mentioned, the authors and the publisher strongly suggest consulting a professional healthcare advisor.

Basic Health Publications, Inc.

Editor: Nancy Ringer
Typesetter/Book design: Gary A. Rosenberg
Cover design: Mike Stromberg

Library of Congress Cataloging-in-Publication Data
Halpern, Georges M.
  The healing trail : essential oils of Madagascar / Georges Halpern, with Peter Weverka.
      p. ; cm.
Includes bibliographical references and index.

      ISBN 978-1-59120-016-1 (Pbk.)
      ISBN 978-1-68162-807-3 (Hardcover)

   1. Essences and essential oils—Madagascar. 2. Aromatherapy.
   [DNLM: 1. Aromatherapy—Madagascar—Popular Works. 2. Oils, Volatile—therapeutic use—Madagascar—Popular Works.
3. Phytotherapy—methods—Madagascar—Popular Works. 4. Plant Extracts—therapeutic use—Madagascar—Popular Works. 5. Plants, Medicinal—Madagascar—Popular Works. WB 925 H195h 2002]
I. Weverka, Peter. II. Title.
RS182.M28 H35   2003
615'.321—dc21   2002154322

Contents

Introduction, 1

1. The Naturalist's Promised Land, 7

2. Introducing Essential Oils and Aromatherapy, 29

3. *Calophyllum Inophyllum* (Foraha Oil), 43

4. Ravintsara, 51

5. Geranium, 57

6. Sweet Basil, 65

7. Cinnamon, 73

8. Ginger, 91

9. Ylang-Ylang, 105

10. Vanilla, 111

11. *Centella asiatica*, 125

12. Biodiversity—Preserving the Rainforest, 131

13. The Healing Trail, 139

    Appendix A. Obtaining Essential Oils from Madagascar, 141

    Appendix B. Traveling to Madagascar, 143

    Notes, 147

    Index, 161

Introduction

This book was written for the purpose of introducing essential oils from Madagascar to aromatherapists and other health-care practitioners who use essential oils in their work. As Chapter 1 explains in detail, Madagascar may be the last remnant of the ancient continent of Gondwanaland. For 85 million years, the flora and fauna of Madagascar evolved in isolation from the rest of the world. Today, eight of ten plants on the island grow there and nowhere else. The plants from which Malagasy essential oils are made benefit by being cultivated in such a unique environment. The island's pristine environment, history of producing essential oils, and ecological diversity make its essential oils distinctive and exceptional; they stand apart from oils produced elsewhere.

We also hope that this book may help prevent ecological damage in Madagascar by bringing Malagasy essential oils to the attention of the world. As you'll read in Chapter 12, the native flora and fauna of Madagascar are disappearing at an alarming rate. They are threatened to such a degree that many consider the island the single highest conservation priority in the world. During the dry season, thousands of square miles of rainforest are shrouded in smoke as Malagasies burn the forest for wood fuel and to clear land for farming and cattle ranching. Today, only a tenth of the island's original rainforests remain. Essential oil production represents a way for the people of Madagascar to earn a living while still preserving the rainforest. By using essential oils from Madagascar, you help conserve the rainforest, its flora, and its fauna.

We have yet another purpose for writing this book—to present Madagascar itself. As visitors will attest, it is easy to fall in love with the island.

It is a fascinating and beautiful country. Throughout this book you will find stories from Malagasy history, portraits of the people who live on Madagascar, and accounts of scientific endeavors undertaken on the island.

EIGHT ESSENTIAL OILS AND A PHARMACEUTICAL EXTRACT

For people who are new to aromatherapy, Chapter 2 explains what essential oils are and how they are used for physical and psychological healing. Thereafter, we investigate eight essential oils and one pharmaceutical extract processed from Malagasy plants:

- *Calophyllum inophyllum.* This rich and luxurious opalescent oil, called foraha oil in Madagascar, soothes damaged skin and discourages wrinkles. It is made from the seed of the plant. Compounds from *Calophyllum inophyllum* may be useful against HIV.

- **Ravintsara.** The deep, camphorous oil of the leaf is a popular choice for massage oils. In Chapter 4, we'll unravel the ravintsara and Ravensara mystery and explain why we believe the ravintsara tree is native to Madagascar.

- **Geranium.** The leaf yields a heavy, olive-green oil that has a rosy, slightly sweet, minty fragrance and remarkable staying power. It has anti-inflammatory qualities and is often prescribed for boils, acne, dermatitis, and burns, as well as for dry skin.

- **Sweet basil.** The stimulating, refreshing, uplifting oil of the leaf has a faint licorice aroma and balsamic undertones. It is believed to improve mental concentration and relieve stress. It also is an antimicrobial and is used in food processing to kill bacteria.

- **Cinnamon.** Aromatic, sweet, and warm, Madagascar cinnamon oil has an animated quality and exciting overtones not found in other cinnamon oils. The oil, which is made from both the bark and the leaf, can destroy microbes and bacteria, help prevent stomach ulcers and diabetes, and restrain the growth of fungi and yeasts.

- **Ginger.** Warming, fortifying, antiseptic, spicy, and soft, gingerroot oil is often an ingredient in colognes and toiletry products. It is also useful in cases of motion sickness, nausea, mononucleosis, and the common cold.

- **Ylang-ylang.** This sensuous, flowery, sweet oil induces feelings of languor and calmness, and many believe it to be an aphrodisiac. In Chapter 9, we'll explain the unique manner in which the oil is distilled and how it is graded.

- **Vanilla.** The long-lasting, rich fragrance of vanilla bean essential oil is a perennial favorite. Madagascar has been the leading producer of natural vanilla for the past century. In Chapter 10, we'll recount the fascinating history of vanilla and explain how it is cultivated and cured.

- ***Centella asiatica.*** Pharmaceutical extracts from the leaf of this plant act on collagen to prevent varicose veins and cellulite from forming. The extracts also heal skin wounds and burns and aid against hypertension.

Throughout this book, we present the folklore and history of these plants and, if they're not native to the island, explain how they arrived in Madagascar. You'll learn how the plants are cultivated, harvested, and processed to make essential oils. You'll also find advice for judging the oils' quality and healing power.

A WORD ABOUT THE CLAIMS OF AROMATHERAPISTS

Many claims are made by aromatherapists about the health-giving properties of the essential oils they use. We have endeavored in this book to view these claims skeptically. At the same time, however, we do not want to discount the claims of aromatherapists and perfumers. Aromas *can* trigger forgotten memories. They *can* change a person's mental state. They *can* have a healing and soothing effect on the body and the soul. Nevertheless, essential oils are not pharmaceutical drugs. The oils affect different people in different ways—and sometimes they have no effect at all. What lulls one person into a sense of well-being may quicken the blood of another. What stirs the passions of one man makes the next guy sneeze.

The sense of smell, more than any other sense, is connected intimately with the brain. For this reason, as Chapter 2 explains, the therapeutic effects of essential oils can never be clearly defined, confirmed, or dismissed, because aromatherapy contains a very strong psychological component. Before we can make clear-cut claims about the value of an essential oil, we need to understand what aromatherapists call "the psychology of scent." We need to know more about how the chemicals in essential oils affect the body and all its systems. To date, much of that information is lacking.

In writing this book, we were faced with a dilemma. Do we describe the claims that aromatherapy makes for these essential oils even though some of the claims are not confirmed by scientific data? Do we ignore these claims entirely? Because the essential oils we present in this book have been revered for centuries for their healing powers, we decided to come down on the side of the aromatherapists; we report what aromatherapists and traditional healers of Madagascar and other places have to say about these essential oils. But we also look forward to a time when essential oils receive the same scrutiny as other medicines. Aromatherapy will come into its own as a healing practice only when more attention is paid to how essential oils—and the different chemicals found in the oils—affect the body.

IN DEFENSE OF SCIENTIFIC STUDIES FROM THE EAST

Throughout this book, we present data from both Eastern and Western scientific studies and experiments. Some in the West have been quick to criticize scientific data from the East (namely China, India, and Japan), but we believe that this kind of criticism is unwarranted. The methods used in the East may vary from those in the West, but the scientists uphold rigorous standards and undertake their studies in the spirit of honest inquiry. They follow sophisticated scientific protocols. The studies we present in this book have been subjected to peer review by panels of international scientists.

MALAGASY NAMES

In writing this book, we were faced with the challenge of Malagasy place names. Since gaining independence from France, the Malagasies have endeavored to recover the ancient names of their cities and towns. Names imposed by the French and other foreign powers have been dropped in favor of the original names. The Malagasies, of course, have every right to decide for themselves what their cities and towns are called, but the original names pose a problem for anyone who studies Madagascar because most of the existing literature refers to the French-imposed names, not the original ones. Taolañaro, for example, is almost always called Fort

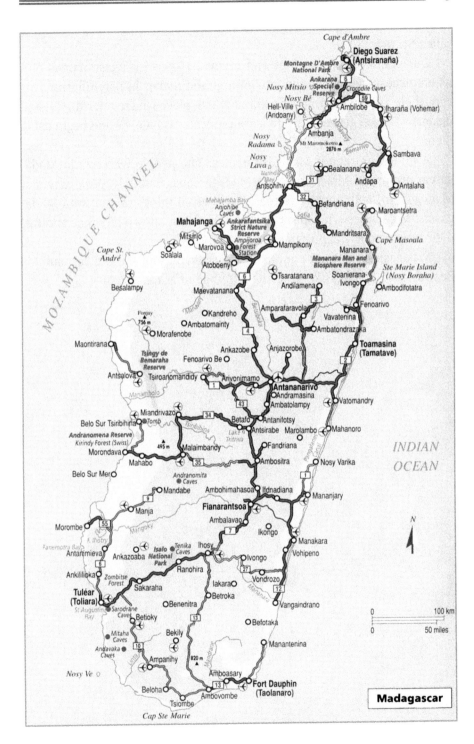

Madagascar

Dauphin. Antsiranana is inevitably called Diégo Suarez. Nosy Boraha is called St. Mary's Island.

Our policy is to call cities and towns by their Malagasy names but, where necessary, to give the foreign-imposed names in parentheses. This way, there will be no confusion about which place we are referring to, and readers will also get a chance to learn the Malagasy names and begin using them.

A final word about Malagasy names: The people who live in Madagascar are called Malagasies, not Madagascans. Similarly, *Malagasy*, not *Madagascan*, is the adjective that describes all things of and from Madagascar. Malagasies who speak English have been known to wince and furl their brows upon hearing the word *Madagascan*.

Malagasies call their country Madagasikara, and the official name is Repoblikan'i Madagasikara, or the Republic of Madagascar.

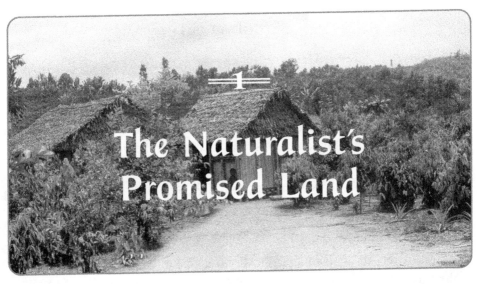

The Naturalist's Promised Land

Madagascar is located in the southwest corner of the Indian Ocean, about 250 miles across the Mozambique Channel from the African mainland. The island is huge. At 1,000 miles in length and 350 miles in width, Madagascar is the fourth largest island in the world (only Greenland, Borneo, and New Guinea are larger). It is roughly the size of Texas and twice the size of Britain. If you were to lay the island across the United States with the southernmost tip on San Diego, the northernmost tip would lie in the middle of Montana.

Madagascar is sometimes called a continent in miniature or the eighth continent because its flora and fauna stand apart from plant and animal species found elsewhere. Because the island has been geographically isolated for so long from the rest of the world, its native flora and fauna evolved according to their own rules. Eight of ten plants that grow in Madagascar grow only on the island. Madagascar has one of the highest rates of endemism—the existence of plant or animal species in only one restricted geographical area—on the planet. The island's plants and animals give a glimpse of what the world looked like 85 million years ago.

Whether or not Madagascar qualifies as a continent, it is most certainly a botanical treasure. Writing in 1771, the French botanist Philibert de Commerson said of Madagascar, "What an admirable country is Madagascar. It deserves not an itinerant observer but entire academies. Madagascar is truly the naturalist's promised land. Here nature seems to have withdrawn into a private sanctuary in order to work in designs which are different from those she has created elsewhere. At every step you are met by the most bizarre and wonderful forms."

WHY CHOOSE ESSENTIAL OILS FROM MADAGASCAR?

For a variety of reasons, essential oils made from plants grown in Madagascar have an excellent reputation among aromatherapists, perfumers, and food-industry chemists. Madagascar's pristine environment, its history as a producer of essential oils, and its ecological diversity have made Malagasy essential oils unique. And there is another compelling reason for using essential oils from Madagascar—doing so helps preserve the rainforest and the animals that live there.

The Pristine Environment

Unfortunately for its people, Madagascar is one of the poorest nations on the earth, with a per capita income of $250 and an external debt of $4 billion. The island is underdeveloped. Because of its poverty, its size, and its difficult terrain, not to mention heavy rainfall in parts of the island, Madagascar's roads and railways are in a constant state of disrepair. Transporting goods and agricultural products from place to place can be extremely difficult. Except around the capital city Antananarivo and a few seaports, industry is lacking in Madagascar. Woeful mismanagement and corruption on the part of government officials, as well as the island's colonial status under France, held back development. Geography is also to blame for Madagascar's poverty. The island is located quite literally at the end of the world. It is far from the centers of commerce and trade. Especially since the opening of the Suez Canal in 1869, which reduced maritime traffic around the Cape of Good Hope, ships do not call often in Malagasy ports.

But the island's underdevelopment and lack of industry has an upside, at least where the production of essential oils is concerned. Madagascar's environment is one of the cleanest and most pristine in the world. The heavy metals and toxins that pollute the topsoil of other countries are rarely found in the soil of Madagascar. Very few of the country's farmers use chemical fertilizers, pesticides, or herbicides, because they can't afford them. Most rivers and streams in Madagascar are free of chemical residues and industrial pollutants. Automobiles are rarely seen outside the capital. Air pollution and the toxins that accompany it—most notably nitrogen oxide and sulfur dioxide—are virtually unknown on the island.

It is hardly necessary to certify whether plants are grown organically in Madagascar. The island is in many ways a throwback to the period before the industrial revolution when the byproducts of industry had yet to pollute fields and streams and modern farming techniques had yet to introduce unnatural substances to the soil. In Madagascar, plants are grown organically by default. Producers of essential oils can be certain that the plants they acquire in Madagascar are pure, uncontaminated, and clean.

The Island's History of Producing Essential Oils

Whatever the demerits of French colonial rule, Madagascar enjoyed some economic advantages from its long association with France. The French policy of maximizing the development of natural resources throughout its empire had the effect of introducing many plants of economic value to Madagascar. The French established, among others, ylang-ylang, cinnamon, niaouli, sweet basil, palmarosa, pepper, ginger, clove, combava, lemongrass, *Calophyllum inophyllum,* and patchouli in Madagascar. Their biggest success was vanilla. As Chapter 10 explains, French horticulturalists introduced vanilla to Madagascar in 1843, and Madagascar subsequently became—and still remains—the world's leading producer of natural vanilla.

As early as the mid-eighteenth century, French botanists Pierre Sonnerat, Philibert de Commerson, Pierre Poivre, and André Michaux were shipping aromatic and medicinal plants from Madagascar to the famous Jardin des Pamplemousses in nearby Mauritius. This botanical park—a portion of the original park, now a tourist attraction, may be visited near Port Louis—served as an experimental station for plants collected in Madagascar, Mauritius, the Comoro Islands, and Réunion, the four French possessions in the southwest Indian Ocean. Throughout the nineteenth century, traffic in plants between the four islands was so brisk that today botanists sometimes have trouble determining which island a plant species came from originally.

In 1897, General Joseph-Simon Galliéni, the first governor general of Madagascar, established the 70-acre Ivoloina botanical park near Taomasina (Tamatave). The park, which still receives visitors today, was modeled after the Jardin des Pamplemousses. It was set up for the experimental cultivation of indigenous and introduced plants. Plants arriving from as far away as the Philippines and the Museum of Natural History in Paris were studied for their economic value and, in some cases, distributed to different parts of the island for cultivation. As a result of this program and others like it, Madagascar became an important exporter of essential oils as early as the 1920s. In 1925, for example, Madagascar exported 2.78 tons of clove oil, 11.7 tons of lemongrass oil, 52 kilograms of patchouli oil, 0.8 tons of geranium oil, 12.8 tons of ylang-ylang oil, and an additional 16.3 tons of miscellaneous oils. The skills needed to cultivate these plants and create these oils have been refined through the decades and handed down from generation to generation.

The Island's Ecological Diversity

In the popular imagination, Madagascar is a tropical island, but within its 225,000 square miles (587,000 square kilometers) can be found many distinct geographical regions where different species of plants grow and can be cultivated. The island has a north-south orientation and extends from 12° to 25° south latitude. It is so long that the Tropic of Capricorn crosses it; its southernmost tip lies in the temperate zone. Madagascar contains humid rainforests and arid deserts, mountain ranges, a vast central plateau, and many subclimates in between. Because the island possesses so much ecological diversity, most medicinal and aromatic plants used in aromatherapy can be grown in one region or another.

On the east side, facing the Indian Ocean, is a humid narrow coastal plain that stretches the length of the island. Here are some of the densest tropical forests in the world, with a canopy lower than is found anywhere else, as well as secondary forests, known as *sàvoka,* where the fan-shaped travelers tree (known in Malagasy as the *ravenala* tree) grows. To the west of the coastal plain, a steep escarpment rises to mountain ranges that run like a backbone from north to south. The escarpment and mountains—the highest mountain, Mount Maromokotro, is 9,436 feet (2,876 meters) above sea level—serve as a buffer against the moist trade winds and monsoon weather of the Indian Ocean. The steep ravines and gullies of the eastern lands are the most inaccessible parts of Madagascar. The area is characterized by high-density rainforest, narrow rivers, and numerous waterfalls.

In the center of the island, like a tilted tabletop, is a high plateau that gradually descends to the Mozambique Channel on the west side. The plateau was once a patchwork of rainforest, brush, and grassland, but it has been almost entirely deforested and is now defaced by *lavaka,* the deep scars left by erosion. The climate on the plateau is temperate. In the south is the Spiny Desert, an arid region that is home to the baobab tree and a variety of thorny cactuslike plants. It bears a superficial resemblance to the American Southwest.

The soil of the high plateau contains a high percentage of laterite, an iron-rich residual product of rock decay that turns the soil red. The red soil, in turn, creates red silt in Malagasy rivers. Ancient sailors nicknamed Madagascar "the great red island" on account of the red silt in its rivers. Due to overgrazing by cattle and the diminishment of the rainforest, rivers on the west side of the island are filled with red silt from the lateritic soil. One river in particular, the Betsiboka, stains the Mozambique Channel for many miles with its red silt. Astronauts orbiting the earth have remarked on the red ocean water around Madagascar, saying that it appeared as though Madagascar was bleeding.

PRESERVING THE RAINFOREST

As Chapter 12 explains in detail, the rainforests of Madagascar are in grave danger. The island's population of 16 million people is increasing by 2.8 percent annually and is expected to double by the year 2025. As the population increases, tracts of rainforest are burned to make new farmland and to provide wood fuel. Only 10 to 20 percent of the original, first-growth rainforest remains, most of it on the inaccessible eastern side of the island. Of the remaining old-growth forest, only 2 percent has been set aside in national parks and nature reserves. Habitat for exotic animals such as lemurs, tenrecs, tree lizards, and forest cuckoos is quickly disappearing. We can only speculate about how many wildlife species and plants are being lost to deforestation in Madagascar.

Essential oils can be an important tool for environmental protection and preservation in Madagascar. The oils represent a way for the island to exploit its floral wealth without damaging the ancient forests. Madagascar lacks the infrastructure to become an industrialized country but, fortunately, has no shortage of fertile land. There is no shortage of water, either, nor a need to build irrigation canals. Most Malagasies agree that the keys to economic prosperity are ecotourism and sustainable agricultural development. The production of essential oils fits very neatly into this long-term economic plan. By purchasing essential oils from Madagascar, you help preserve the rainforest, its plants, and the many animals that make their home there.

MADAGASCAR: THE LAST REMNANT OF GONDWANALAND?

Previous to the discovery of continental drift and the theory of plate tectonics, scientists were at a loss to explain why the same plant genera and plant and animal fossils could be found in widely separated geographical regions. Botanists, for example, have identified twenty-six plant genera that are found exclusively in Madagascar and South America. One of them, *Ravenala* (Musaceae), is found only in Madagascar, Brazil, and Guiana. Fossils of certain tropical plants have been found on the Arctic island of Spitsbergen. These anomalies seem to contradict Darwin's theory of evolution, which holds that species derive from a common ancestor. How could species originate from the same ancestor if they are found oceans apart?

In the nineteenth century, scientists explained this puzzle by proposing that submerged land bridges and continents once linked faraway lands. To explain why lemurs are found in Madagascar and lemurlike bush babies and lorises are found, respectively, in Africa and India, English zoologist Philip Lutley Sclater proposed the existence in the Indian Ocean of a sunken continent called Lemuria. In the April 1864 edition of *The Quarterly Journal of Science*, a publication of the Zoological Society of London, Sclater wrote:

> To conclude therefore, granted the hypothesis of the derivative origin of species, the anomalies of the Mammal-fauna of Madagascar can best be explained by supposing that, anterior to the existence of Africa in its present shape, a large continent occupied parts of the Atlantic and Indian Ocean stretching out towards (what is now) America on the west, and to India and its islands on the east; that this continent was broken up into islands, of which some became amalgamated with the present continent of Africa, and some possibly with what is now Asia—and that in Madagascar and the Mascarene Islands [Réunion, Mauritius, and Rodrigues] we have existing relics of the great continent, for which . . . I should propose the name Lemuria!

The continent of Lemuria, named for Madagascar's cutest and most famous primate, subsequently took on a life of its own under the direction of naturalists, Theosophists, occultists, and assorted psychics. In the 1880s, German naturalist Ernst Heinrich Haeckel suggested that fossils of early humans had not been discovered because humans developed on the submerged continent of Lemuria. "Sclater has given this continent the name of Lemuria," he wrote, "from the semi-apes which were characteristic of it." Haeckel was the champion of evolution in the German-speaking world. His books were widely read, influencing, among others, the founder of Theosophy, Helena Petrovna Blavatsky, who took up the cause of Lemuria in *The Secret Doctrine* (1888). Blavatsky claimed that Lemuria extended into the Atlantic as well as the Indian Ocean and was occupied by a race of four-armed, egg-laying hermaphrodites. Another Theosophist, William Scott-Elliot, put the continent in the Atlantic, Indian, and Pacific Oceans in his *The Lost Lemuria* (1904). Scott-Elliot's Lemurians were 12 to 15 feet tall and kept dinosaurs as pets. In *Lemuria: The Lost Continent of the Pacific* (1931), Wishar Cerve has Californians entering Lemuria by way of a hidden, jewel-encrusted cave inside Mount Shasta. The occultist Edgar Cayce found the Garden of Eden in Lemuria during one of his psychic journeys. The 35,000-year-old spirit-warrior Ramtha also hails from Lemuria, according to medium J. Z. Knight, author of *I Am Ramtha* (1986), who hears and sometimes transcribes Ramtha's voice for the benefit of her readers.

While psychics and occultists were exploring the lost continent of Lemuria, a German scientist named Alfred Wegener set about tackling the problem of why the same fossils and plants are found on different continents. Wegener noticed that the coastlines of Africa and South America appear to fit like pieces of a jigsaw puzzle and that identical Mesosaurus fossils are found on both of those continents. Geographical features on different continents, he noticed, sometimes match one another when the continents are brought together. The Appalachian Mountains and Scottish Highlands, for example, have the same distinctive rock strata. From this and other evidence, Wegener formulated the theory of continental drift in 1924. He believed that the continents were originally compressed into a protocontinent called Pangaea (the word means "all lands" in Greek) that rifted or split apart to form the continents we know today.

Continental drift was rejected by the scientific community because it failed to explain how the continents managed to drift. In the 1950s, however, oceanographers discovered something that gave credence to Wegener's theory: ridges and trenches on the ocean floor. These ridges and trenches are formed by moving tectonic plates. Wegener's theory of continental drift was folded into a grander theory called plate tectonics. According to this theory, the continents and ocean floor rest on tectonic plates that float on a layer of heated rock below the earth's crust. Because tectonic plates float, they drift. Where they collide, mountain ranges are formed. Where they move apart, hot molten lava seeps from below the earth's crust to form ridges. The north-south Mid-Atlantic Ridge, the divergent-plate boundary that runs like a seam across the floor of the Atlantic Ocean, is one such ridge.

Tectonic forces split Pangaea into two continents, Laurasia and Gondwanaland, at the end of the Paleozoic era 200 to 250 million years ago. Gondwanaland became what are now the continents of the southern hemisphere, as well as India. In the mid- to late-Jurassic period, about 165 million years ago, Madagascar and India—they formed a mini-continent called Greater India—split from Africa and began drifting into the Indian Ocean. Approximately 85 million years ago, India and Madagascar parted company. India "slammed" into Asia in a violent slow-motion collision that produced the Himalaya Mountains. Madagascar has been on its own for at least 85 million years. The lemurs of Madagascar, the bush babies of Africa, and the lorises of Asia share a common ancestor who lived not on the lost continent of Lemuria but on Gondwanaland.

Gondwanaland became South America, Africa, Madagascar, India, and Australia. Most of these landmasses border other lands, whereas Madagascar was isolated for 85 million years. Its flora and fauna evolved in a time capsule. Is Madagascar the last remnant of the ancient continent Gondwanaland? It is intriguing to think so.

THE BOTANICAL TREASURE-HOUSE

Madagascar has one of the richest and most varied flora in the world. Although the island accounts for only 2 percent of the African continent, 20 percent of the vascular plant species in Africa are found in Madagascar. (Vascular plants, which comprise the majority of plants, have specialized tissues for moving water and photosynthetic products. Algae and mosses are nonvascular plants.) Fully 80 percent of its vascular plant species are endemic. In other words, eight of ten vascular plant species on the island are found in Madagascar and nowhere else in the world.

Madagascar is a botanical treasure-house. Estimating the number of plant species on the island is in itself difficult, because remote areas of the island have not been explored by botanists. The number of plant species ranges from 7,300 to 14,000. To put these numbers in perspective, Brazil, the leader in plant species diversity, has about 55,000 plant species. However, Brazil is eleven times larger than Madagascar. Moreover, Brazil has no endemic plant families, while Madagascar has ten. Other statistics that give a picture of Madagascar's botanical diversity and uniqueness include the following:

- Ten plant families and 260 genera are endemic to Madagascar. Only Australia, with 13 endemic plant families, has more endemic plant families than Madagascar, and Australia is 13 times the size of Madagascar.

- More than 1,000 species of endemic orchids are found on Madagascar. This total exceeds the number found in all of Africa.

- More bamboo species are found in the Tsaratanana Massif, a mountain range in northern Madagascar, than in all of Africa.

- More than 130 species of palms are found on the island, far more than are found in all of Africa.

These statistics are startling, and they underscore the importance of saving Madagascar's rainforest. We simply do not know how many undiscovered plant species are being made extinct by fire, erosion, and other forms of environmental degradation. About 50 percent of pharmaceutical drugs are derived from plants. Who knows if another rosy periwinkle (*Catharanthus roseus*) is waiting to be discovered in Madagascar? As Chapter 12 explains, pharmaceutical drugs derived from the rosy periwinkle, also known as the Madagascar periwinkle, have dramatically improved patients' chances of recovering from childhood leukemia and Hodgkin's disease.

A Word about Madagascar's Fauna and Megafauna

Although this book concerns Madagascar's flora, no book about Madagascar is complete without a word about its fauna as well. Like the plants, the animals of Madagascar evolved in isolation from the rest of the world. Ninety percent of the island's 260 reptile species are endemic. Two-thirds of the world's chameleon species live in Madagascar, leading some researchers to believe that the chameleon evolved first on the island. The island boasts forty species of tenrec, the primitive animal that resembles a mole. Madagascar's lemurs are known to everybody, but few know that thirty-three species of lemur live on the island. Twenty-one percent of the world's primates are found in Madagascar. For the purposes of study, primatologists—the scientists who study monkeys, apes, and gorillas—divide the world into four regions, with Madagascar being a region unto itself (the other regions are South and Central America, Southeast Asia, and mainland Africa). Interestingly, Madagascar's animals do not exhibit the same fear of humans that is found on the African mainland, most likely because humans arrived so late in Madagascar. Visitors to the island's national parks and forest reserves can approach the animals and observe them from short distances.

Because Madagascar was one of the last landmasses on earth to be occupied by people, its megafauna were among the last to be hunted to extinction. *Megafauna* are extraordinary large animals such as the woolly mammoth, the moa of New Zealand, the big flightless geese of Hawaii, and the Harrington's mountain goat (*Oreamnos harrintoni*) and giant sloth of North America. Hunter-gatherers took up agriculture in part because they exhausted their supply of protein-rich megafauna. Whereas the extinction of the megafauna in North America, for example, took place at about 10,000 B.C.E., the large animals were still living in Madagascar as late as 1300 C.E., when humans settled the high plateau. A visitor to the high plateau in of Madagascar in 1300 C.E. might have encountered:

- **The giant lemur.** There were 17 species of giant lemur, with the largest the size of a mountain gorilla.

- **The flightless aepyornis.** This 1,000-pound, 10-foot-tall bird resembled the ostrich. Its eggs, which are about 18 inches tall, are still found on the island. Aepyornis is also known as the "elephant bird" because it was supposed to be strong enough to lift an elephant.

- **The kilopilopitsofy.** This hippolike animal had large, floppy ears. Unconfirmed sightings, the most recent in 1976, still occur on the island.

- **The pygmy hippo.** The pygmy hippo was a scaled-down version of the full-size hippos found on the African mainland. The last sightings occurred in the nineteenth century.

Perhaps the most amazing member of Madagascar's megafauna is a fish, the steel-blue coelacanth (sē'-lə-kanth). Ichthyologists—zoologists who specialize in the study of fish—proclaimed the fish extinct, but the six-foot-long, 150-pound, heavily scaled fish went right on swimming in the Indian Ocean without any regard for ichthyology. In 1952, a coelacanth was caught in the waters between Madagascar and the Comoro Islands, and its "extinct" status was revoked. The species is believed to be 60 to 75 million years old, predating the dinosaurs. The *Encyclopedia Britannica* of 1960 says about the fish, "The coelacanth has lived the longest with the least change of form." Our fingers are crossed in the hope that the aepyornis, giant lemur, and pigmy hippo will reappear in Madagascar after the manner of the coelacanth.

A BRIEF HISTORY OF MADAGASCAR

Madagascar's people came from mainland Africa, from Arabia, and, astonishingly, from Indonesia, all the way across the Indian Ocean. The island's sixteen tribes sometimes lived in peace and sometimes didn't. The island was briefly a haven for pirates, and for 65 years it was a colony of France. And if you'd care to know more about the past of this fascinating country, read on.

Early History

According to Malagasy mythology, the island was first inhabited by a tribe of pale dwarflike people called the Vazimba. Some believe that the Vazimba still inhabit the deepest recesses of the forest. The Malagasy practice ancestor worship, and the Vazimba are venerated as the most ancient of ancestors. The kings of some Malagasy tribes claim blood kinship to the Vazimba.

Archeologists place the arrival of humans on Madagascar between 200 and 500 c.e., making the island one of the last landmasses to be occupied by humans. These first inhabitants were seafarers from Southeast Asia, probably Borneo or the southern Celebes. They came to the island as part of the great Austronesian expansion, the movement of people that populated the Malay Peninsula, Java, Sumatra, New Zealand, and all of Polynesia and Micronesia, as well as Hawaii and the Easter Islands. No evidence exists to suggest that the Bantus of nearby Africa populated Madagascar before the Austronesians. It appears that the first inhabitants of

Madagascar came in outrigger canoes directly across the Indian Ocean from Indonesia, a journey of 3,700 miles made possible by trade winds and the equatorial east-west current. The anthropologist Jared Diamond writes about the Austronesian expansion to Madagascar:

> These Austronesians, with their Austronesian language and modi-
> fied Austronesian culture, were already established on Madagascar
> by the time it was first visited by Europeans, in 1500. This strikes
> me as the single most astonishing fact of human geography for the
> entire world. It's as if Columbus, on reaching Cuba, had found it
> occupied by blue-eyed, blond-haired Scandinavians speaking a lan-
> guage close to Swedish, even though the nearby North American
> continent was inhabited by Native Americans speaking Amerindi-
> an languages. How on earth could prehistoric people from Borneo,
> presumably voyaging on boats without maps or compasses, end up
> in Madagascar?

In their technology and agriculture, Malagasies share many traits with Indonesians. Techniques of rice cultivation are the same in both places. A visitor to the central highlands of Madagascar, gazing at the rice paddies, might think he or she is in a Southeast Asian country. Like the Indonesians, the Malagasies use outrigger-style canoes (the outrigger canoe, with its pontoon, represented a major advancement over the dugout canoe, which is difficult to balance and incapable of long ocean voyages). Both cultures practice ancestor worship and believe that the dead influence the living. Unlike their neighbors on the African continent, who favor round huts, Malagasies live in four-cornered dwellings. They used two-valved bellows—an invention of the Malay Peninsula—to forge iron. They dressed in cloth woven of vegetable fibers or raffia (a fabric made from the stripped membranes of the raffia palm), not animal skins or wool, as did Africans and Europeans.

The Merina tribe—the name means "People of the Land of Wide Prospects"—is the largest in Madagascar, and its people bear a striking resemblance to Indonesians. Looking at a member of the Merina tribe, you might think you were looking at a native of Jakarta. The Merina, however, are but one of Madagascar's sixteen tribes (the Malagasies do not object to the term "tribe" or find it pejorative). Other tribes have the dark skin and solid stature of Bantus from the African mainland. Still others have an Arabic cast. Most are of mixed racial stock. Today's Madagascar is an amalgam of different races and cultural influences—Southeast Asian, African, Arabic, Indian, and French. Perhaps because Madagascar is an island and the people who settled there had to cut ties with the places from whence they came, all Malagasies, no matter their ethnic origin, speak the same language: Malagasy, a language that belongs to the Indonesian branch of the Malayan-Polynesian linguistic group. Malagasies are fortunate to all speak the same language. A common language is one reason why they have been spared the fierce ethnic divisions that sometimes tear apart other African countries.

The Merina, who are thought to be the descendents of those early Indonesian seafarers and the source of the Malagasy language, make their home in the central plateau of Madagascar. However, archeologists and linguists speculate that the Merina lived for many centuries on the coasts of Madagascar. (Archeological records show no evidence of anyone living in the central plateau until the thirteenth century.) As new settlers arrived, they adopted the language of the Merina tribe. When eventually the Merina migrated to the central plateau, their language was well established on the coasts.

Madagascar as Myth and Legend

Unfortunately, scholars have neglected the ancient trade routes of the Indian Ocean, so little is known about them, and it is hard to say when or whether traders visited Madagascar previous to the second millennium. Still, ancient mariners very likely were familiar with Madagascar; the island is described in both Arabic and European myths and legends. To medieval Arab navigators and geographers, the very large island off the southern coast of Ophir (Africa) was known by various names: Phebol, Cernea, Menuthias, Medruthis, Sherbezat, Camarcada, and the Island of the Moon. Some have suggested that the Roc in the tale of Sinbad the Sailor, found in *The Book of a Thousand and One Nights,* was the flightless aepyornis.

Madagascar received its name from none other than Marco Polo, the fourteenth-century Italian explorer. Writing his memoirs in a Pisan prison, Marco Polo described an African island of untold wealth called "Madeigascar." The Italian explorer heard about the island secondhand during his travels in Asia. Most scholars believe that he was writing about Mogadishu, the port located in present-day Somalia. Nevertheless, the name *Mada-*

gascar was attached to the island by Italian cartographers during the Renaissance, and it stuck. Previous to the name imposed by Europeans, the Malagasies knew their island as *Nosin-dambo*, "The Land of Wild Boars"; *Izao rehetra izao*, "This All"; and *Izao tontolo izao*, "This Whole."

Bantus, Arabs, and Luckless Europeans

The closer you come to the coasts of Madagascar, the more people resemble the Bantus of mainland Africa rather than Indonesians. Bantu settlers probably crossed the Mozambique Channel to Madagascar at the same time as, or shortly after, the Indonesians arrived. Although the majority of words in the Malagasy language are of Malayan-Polynesian origin, a smattering of Bantu words—*omby* (ox), *ondry* (sheep), and others—is spoken as well. Some anthropologists cite these Bantu words as evidence that Indonesian and Bantu settlers intermixed quite early in the island's history.

The Bantus brought with them the gourdlike *jejolava* and multistringed *valiha*, the musical instruments on which distinctive Malagasy music is played. The Bantus also brought a cultural trait that is peculiar to East Africa, not to mention Texas and Argentina—an obsession with cattle. Especially on the southern savannahs of Madagascar, where African influences are strongest, wealth and social status are measured in cattle. Here, the huge, humpbacked, lyre-horned zebus outnumber the inhabitants two or three to one. In addition to being a source of food, the zebus represent a link between the living and the dead. No important event—a harvest, wedding, or funeral—is complete without the sacrifice of a zebu to appease the ancestors and obtain their blessings.

Beginning in the tenth or eleventh century, Arabic and Zanzibari traders working their way down the east coast of Africa in their dhows (boats) established settlements on the west coast of Madagascar. These newcomers were slave traders. Arriving with textiles and iron goods, they departed with human chattel for the Arabian Peninsula. Their descendants formed the Antaimoro tribe, which today lives on the southeast coast near to Manakara. Although Arab immigrants were few in number compared to the Indonesians and Bantus, they left a lasting impression on the culture of Madagascar. The Malagasy names for seasons, months, days, and coins are Arabic in origin. So is the practice of circumcision, the communal grain pool, and different forms of salutation. The Arab magicians, known as the *ombiasy*, established themselves in the courts of many Malagasy tribal kingdoms. And the Arabs introduced the concept of *vintana,* or destiny, which is central to Malagasy thinking. In his excellent book *The Eighth Continent,* Peter Tyson writes of *vintana:*

> This idea, the most significant Arab contribution to Malagasy culture, is simply that everyone, by virtue of the date and time of his or her birth, inherits a particular destiny. In may be a lucky one (*tsara*) or an unlucky one (*ratsy*). Either way, it is one's for life and must be taken into consideration when planning all major events, such as getting married or building a tomb. Though the laws of *vintana* are eternal and unchangeable, an ombiasy in some cases may be able to reverse a bad destiny through a complex process of divination.

Although the first Arabic traders to settle in Madagascar were almost certainly devout followers of Islam—the Antaimoro tribe claims ancestry from Mecca, and Mahilaka, one of the oldest archeological sites in Madagascar, contains a large mosque—their modern-day descendants do not practice the Islamic faith. The 7 percent of Malagasies who practice Islam are recent immigrants from the Comoro Islands. Before it was forsaken, however, Islam imposed the patriarchal system of family and clan rule on Madagascar. Previous to the Arab immigration, the Malagasies practiced the Polynesian matriarchal system whereby rights of privilege and property are conferred equally on men and women.

By the fifteenth century, Europeans had wrested the spice trade from the Muslims. They did so by sidestepping the Middle East and sending their cargo ships around the Cape of Good Hope to India. A Portuguese mariner named Diogo Dias became the first European to set foot on Madagascar when his ship, bound for India, blew off course in 1500. In the ensuing two hundred years, the English and French tried and failed to establish settlements on the island. Fever, dysentery, hostile Malagasy tribesmen, and the trying arid climate of southern Madagascar terminated the English settlement near Toliary (Tuléar) in 1646, just a year after its founding. An English settlement in Nosy Bé, in the north, came to the same end at its own one-year anniversary in 1649.

The French colony at Taolañaro (Fort Dauphin) fared a little better. It lasted thirty years. On Christmas night 1672, local Antanosy tribesmen, perhaps angry because fourteen French soldiers in the fort had recently divorced their Malagasy wives to marry fourteen orphan French women who had been sent out to the colony, massacred the fourteen grooms and thirteen of the fourteen brides. The Antanosy then besieged the Taolañaro stockade for eighteen months. A ship of the French East India Company, the *White Pigeon*, rescued the surviving thirty men and one widow in 1674.

Pirates and Slave Traders

Most schoolboys (and a few schoolgirls, too) make their first acquaintance with Madagascar in connection with the island's history as a pirate stronghold. Such pirate luminaries as Captain William Kidd, Henry Every, John Bowen, and Thomas Tew made Madagascar their base of operations between 1680 and 1725. From the safety of Antongil Bay and Nosy Boraha (St. Mary's Island), a small island 12 miles off the northeast coast of Madagascar, the pirates plundered merchant ships in the Indian Ocean, the Red Sea, and the Persian Gulf. The pirates robbed ships bound for Europe of their silks, cloth, spices, and jewels and ships going the opposite direction, to India, of their coin, gold, and silver. They robbed Indian cargo ships trading between ports in the Indian Ocean, as well as ships commissioned by the East India Companies of France, England, and the Netherlands. The pilgrim fleet sailing between Surat in India and Mocha on the tip of the Arabian Peninsula was a favorite target, because the wealthy pilgrims often carried jewels and other finery with them to Mecca. In 1695, Henry Every and his men captured two Indian warships, the *Fateh Mohammed* and the *Ging-i-Saway*, which were ferrying gold and gems worth $200 million. In 1721, John Taylor, Oliver la Buse, and their crews relieved the Portuguese carrack *Nostra Senhora de Cabo* of $400 million in diamonds and other treasure. Merchants in India, various ports of Africa, and Réunion Island were eager to fence the pirates' stolen goods. The low-paid seamen who manned merchant ships in the Indian Ocean seldom put up a fight, having little reason or motivation to risk their lives. The pirates often recruited crewmen from the ships they captured.

Madagascar hosted what has been called the Golden Age of Piracy, with some chroniclers even suggesting that the pirate society on Nosy Boraha was an early, noble experiment in democracy. While it is true that the pirates elected their own officers and enjoyed an egalitarianism that could not be found elsewhere in 1700, it must be remembered that these marauders made their living by robbery and murder on the high seas.

Moreover, their presence in Madagascar, along with that of English and French slave traders, had a devastating effect on the island.

Previous to the arrival of Europeans, the Malagasy tribes had occasionally waged wars to capture and enslave prisoners. The slaves were either sold to Arab traders or kept as laborers. With the arrival of European slave traders, human chattel became more valuable, and the coastal tribes of Madagascar took to warring with each other to obtain prisoners for the lucrative slave trade. (The historian Hugh Thomas reports that Malagasy slaves were prized in the Carolinas for their skill at growing rice.) Instead of using spears and cutlasses, the tribesmen fought with muskets, musket balls, and gunpowder that they obtained from the Europeans. The wars were fierce and brutal. Because of their relationship with the pirates on Nosy Boraha, the Betsimisaraka in eastern Madagascar had more firearms than any other tribe. They overpowered their neighbors, the Antakarana and the Tsimihety, and even raided the Comoro Islands. As the tribe on the west coast with the most connections to the slave trade, the Sakalava also had access to guns and gunpowder and subdued the other tribes on the west coast. Tribal chiefs who failed to capture prisoners for the slave trade sometimes did what had previously been considered unthinkable—they sold their own people into slavery.

The Merina Monarchy

In 1777, an adventurous French trader named Nicolas Mayeur hacked his way up the steep eastern escarpment of Madagascar to see what lay on the other side. In his own words, he discovered "in the center of the island, thirty leagues from the sea, a country, until then unknown, surrounded as it was by wild and savage tribes, with lights, commerce, and an active political organization and administration." Mayeur had found the Merina kingdom. This kingdom of rice farmers had been living in relative isolation from the rest of Madagascar for several centuries, but by 1824 the Merina had conquered nearly all of Madagascar, thanks to the leadership of two shrewd kings, Andrianampoinimerina (circa 1745–1810) and his son Radama I (1792–1828).

By marrying the princesses of different Merina clans and warring against other princes—by making love *and* war—Andrianampoinimerina united the Merina kingdom. He established Antananarivo as the capital of Madagascar and built the royal palace, or *rova*, on a hilltop overlooking the city. The king was ambitious. He proclaimed, *"Ny ranomasina no vala-pariako"* ("the sea is the boundary of my rice field"). But what distinguished Andrianampoinimerina from other ambitious kings and tribal chiefs was his ability to administer. The king codified the laws. He supervised the building of dykes and trenches to increase the amount of arable land around Antananarivo. He introduced the metal spade and compelled rice farmers to use it. King Andrianampoinimerina was an exemplary military commander. By the time of his death in 1810, he had conquered the Bara and Betsileo highland tribes and was preparing to push the boundaries of his kingdom to the shores of the island.

His son Radama I (Radama the Great) assumed the throne during a great turning point in European history that had repercussions even in faraway Madagascar. With the defeat of Napoléon, the balance of power in Europe and the European colonies shifted in England's favor. The English, eager to exert control over the trade routes of the Indian Ocean, captured the islands of Réunion and Mauritius from the French. Although they returned Réunion, they kept Mauritius as a base for expanding the British empire. To woo Madagascar from French control, Mauritius's governor recognized Radama I as king of Madagascar, a diplomatic maneuver meant to underscore the idea that the island was sovereign and therefore unclaimed by any European powers. Radama I signed treaties with England outlawing the slave trade and admitting Protestant missionaries into Madagascar. The terms of these treaties seemed innocuous enough, but the Protestant missionaries, the English knew, would spread British influence as well as Christian charity, and outlawing the slave trade, the English hoped, would weaken Réunion by depriving that island of slave laborers for its sugar plantations. In return for outlawing the slave trade, Madagascar received what the treaty called "The Equivalent": an annual sum of a thousand pounds in gold, another thousand in silver, stated amounts of gun powder, flints, and muskets, plus 400 surplus British Army uniforms. The governor of Mauritius also sent military advisers who accompanied and sometimes led Merina soldiers in their battles against the Sakalava and Betsimisaraka. In 1824, having defeated the Betsimisaraka, Radama I declared, "Today, the whole island is mine! Madagascar has but one master." The king died in 1828 while leading his army on a punitive expedition against the Betsimisaraka.

The thirty-three-year reign of Queen Ranavalona I (Ranavalona the

Cruel), the widow of Radama I, began inauspiciously with the queen murdering the dead king's heir (his nephew) and relatives. She repudiated the treaties that Radama I had signed with Britain. The aristocrats and sorcerers who had lost influence under the liberal regime of the previous two Merina kings reasserted their power during the reign of Ranavalona I. Emerging from a dangerous illness in 1835, the queen credited her recovery to the *sampy*, the twelve talismans endowed with supernatural powers that were housed on the palace grounds. To appease the *sampy* who had restored her health, she issued a royal edict prohibiting the practice of Christianity in Madagascar, expelled British missionaries from the island, and persecuted Christian converts who would not renounce their religion. Christian customs "are not the customs of our ancestors," she explained. The queen scrapped the legal reforms initiated by Andrianampoinimerina and reinstated the old system of trial by ordeal. People suspected of committing crimes—most were tried for the crime of practicing Christianity—were made to drink the poison of the *tangena* tree. If they survived the ordeal, which few did, they were judged innocent. Malagasy Christians would remember this period as *ny tany maizina,* or "the time when the land was dark." By some estimates, 150,000 Christians died during the reign of Ranavalona the Cruel. The island grew more isolated, and commerce with other nations came to a standstill.

Unbeknownst to the queen, her son and heir, crown prince Radama II, attended Roman Catholic masses in secret. The young man grew up under the influence of French nationals in Antananarivo. Either he was extraordinarily naïve or he was desperate to end his mother's despotic regime. In 1854, he wrote a letter to Napoléon III, inviting France to invade Madagascar. On June 28, 1855, he signed the Lambert Charter. This document gave Joseph-François Lambert, an enterprising French businessman who had arrived in Madagascar only three weeks before, the exclusive right to exploit all minerals, forests, and unoccupied land in Madagascar in exchange for a 10 percent royalty to be paid to the Merina monarchy. In years to come, the French would use the Lambert Charter and the prince's letter to Napoléon III to justify the Franco-Hova Wars and the annexation of Madagascar as a colony. In 1857, the queen uncovered a plot by Radama II and French nationals in the capital to remove her from power. She immediately expelled all foreigners from Madagascar. Ranavalona the Cruel died in 1861.

In his brief two years on the throne, King Radama II reopened trade with Mauritius and Réunion, invited Christian missionaries and foreigners to return to Madagascar, and reinstated most of Radama I's reforms. His liberal policies angered the aristocracy, however, and he was strangled in a coup d'état engineered by Rainivoninahitriniony, the prime minister. This cunning man and his equally cunning brother, Rainilaiarivory, would rule Madagascar from behind the scenes for the remaining thirty-two years of the Merina monarchy. First Rainivoninahitriniony and then his brother married Queen Rasoaherina, the widow of Radama II. Rainilaiarivory also married the last two queens of Madagascar, Ranavalona II and Ranavalona III.

In 1869, Queen Ranavalona II, who had been educated by the London Missionary Society, was baptized into the Anglican Episcopal Church and subsequently made that faith the official state religion of Madagascar. The queen had all the *sampy* burned in a public display. Catholic and Protestant missionaries arrived in numbers to build churches and schools. Today, nominally at least, half of Malagasies are Christian, split about evenly between the Catholic and Protestant churches. (It has been said that the Malagasy were "merely vaccinated into Christianity," because their ancient religions are still practiced side by side with Christianity.) The reign of Queen Ranavalona II was the heyday of British influence in Madagascar. In parts of the island, English replaced French as the second language. *Cup, carpet,* and other English words entered the Malagasy language. British arms and troops arrived on the island by way of South Africa. An English colonel named Digby Willoughby (we mention his name because it is so perfectly English) was made head of the army.

Angry because the Lambert Charter had been canceled, and seeking to restore property that had been confiscated from French citizens, France invaded Madagascar in 1883 in what became known as the first Franco-Hova War (*Hova* being the name of the Merina aristocrats). At the war's end, Madagascar ceded Antsiranana (Diégo Suarez) on the northern coast to France and paid 560,000 gold francs to the heirs of Joseph-François Lambert. In Europe, meanwhile, diplomats partitioning the African continent worked out an agreement whereby Britain, to obtain the Sultanate of Zanzibar, ceded its share of Helgoland to Germany and renounced all claims to Madagascar. The agreement spelled doom for Madagascar. Prime Minister Rainilaiarivory had been able to play England and France against each other, but now France could meddle in the affairs of the island without fear of reprisals from England. In 1895, a French flying column landed in Mahajanga (Majunga) and marched by way of the Betsiboka River to Antananarivo. The city's defenders were taken by surprise. They had expected an attack from the much closer east coast. Twenty French soldiers died fighting and six thousand died of malaria and other diseases before the second Franco-Hova War ended with the capture of the capital city. In 1896, the French Parliament voted to annex Madagascar. The 103-year-old Merina monarchy ended, and the royal family was exiled in Algeria.

The French Colony

Under French colonial rule, Madagascar took the good with the bad. The French oversaw the building of roads, railroads, airports, schools, and hospitals. They introduced modern methods of agriculture and stockbreeding. Slavery was abolished once and for all. As explained later in the book, programs for agricultural development were put in place throughout the island. The French policy of relying on local people to manage civic affairs encouraged tribes apart from the Merina to take a hand in governing Madagascar. Forest reserves were established. Laws against indiscriminately burning the rainforest were placed on the books for the first time.

Nevertheless, Malagasies chafed under French rule. By law, all men between the ages of sixteen and sixty were forced to work building roads and public works at low wages for fifty days annually. Under the laws of the *indigénat* (laws imposed on all non-French citizens in France's colonies), French citizens enjoyed rights of association and movement that were denied Malagasies. Only the French language, not Malagasy or English, was permitted in schools. The emphasis on growing crops for export led to food shortages when land that had previously been devoted to rice cultivation was used for growing coffee.

An Independent Madagascar

In March 1947, thousands of Malagasies, many of them veterans of the French army who had served in World War II, revolted against French colonial rule. The French suppression of the three-year revolt was brutal. Conservative estimates put the number of Malagasy dead at 80,000 (the island's population was 3 to 4 million). Ten years later, however, a France eager to shed its colonial empire permitted Madagascar to hold a referendum for independence. The referendum passed, and the Republic of Madagascar was born on June 26, 1960.

Madagascar aligned itself with France and the West in the early years of independence, but in 1975, after three years of coups and political turmoil, the country elected a socialist named Didier Ratsiraka as president. The president's self-styled Christian-Marxist state—Ratsiraka even wrote his own *Boky Mena*, or *Red Book*, after the example of Mao Tse-tung—proved a disaster. French technocrats fled the island and investors shunned it after the president nationalized banks and other institutions.

Madagascar, it has been said, was a victim of the Cold War as a result of its politicians' miscalculations and poor leadership in siding with the Eastern bloc. As the Eastern bloc to which Madagascar aligned itself lost its economic clout, the economy of Madagascar slowly collapsed. It has not recovered. At the time of this publication, however, Madagascar has elected a remarkable young president named Marc Ravalomanana (known locally as Mr. Tiko for a brand of yogurt he made famous). A businessman and former mayor of Antananarivo, Ravalomanana has pledged to follow a free-market path, end government corruption, and open the country to foreign investment. Malagasies are hopeful that their island's economy will soon improve.

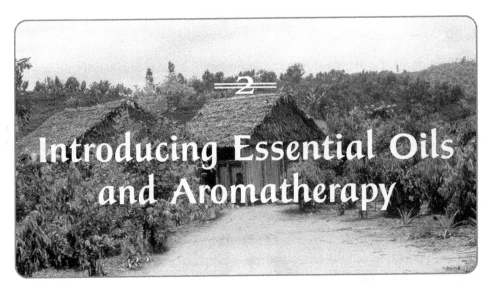

Introducing Essential Oils and Aromatherapy

Aromatherapy is the art and, less frequently, the science of using essential oils from plants to heal the body and the mind. Essential oils were among the first medicines, and in a sense, aromatherapy is a rediscovery of plants' healing power. In their medicine kits, for example, Dioscorides, Pliny, and other renowned physicians of ancient times carried three essential oils we describe in this book—cinnamon, sweet basil, and gingerroot. They applied these oils to their patients in the form of compresses, balms, and unguents (healing salves).

Today, essential oils are used for a variety of purposes in addition to healing, including the manufacture of household cleaners, detergents, pharmaceuticals, and nutriceuticals. They are also blended into cosmetics, lotions, skin-care products, soaps, toothpastes, and shampoos. Essential oil production is a $700 million per year industry, and worldwide annual production of essential oils amounts to about 45,000 tons.

When you bend over to smell a rose, linger by the door of a bakery, or inhale the bouquet of Château Lynch-Bages 1982, you are practicing a primitive form of aromatherapy. Certain aromas awaken the senses. They relax the body and impart a sense of well-being. Skilled aromatherapists know how to blend essential oils to calm the nerves, increase circulation, quicken the mind, excite sexual longing, or do any number of other things to improve their patients' mental and physical health.

WHAT IS AN ESSENTIAL OIL?

The essential oil, it has been said, is the heart and soul of a plant. It gives a plant its scent and may also repel insects, attract bees and wasps for fertilization of the plant's flowers, and protect the plant against decay, fungal infestations, bacteria, and mold. Some of the same essential oil properties that serve plants in nature also provide health benefits to humans. Food manufacturers, for example, sometimes include essential oils in their products as a way of preventing bacterial growth. The oils are purer and more healthful than chemical antibacterial agents, such as chlorine. Many skin-care products also make use of antibacterial essential oils. In nature, these oils protect plants against bacteria, and they do the same for us when rubbed on the skin.

Essential oil molecules consist of carbon, hydrogen, and oxygen atoms. The application of heat releases these molecules from plants, thereby producing a fragrance. The oils are volatile; when an essential oil is exposed to air, its aroma characteristics immediately begin to change.

Essential oil is extracted through a variety of methods from the cellular glands, or sacs, of a plant's leaves, flowers, stems, twigs, seeds, roots, rind, fruit, or bark, and sometimes from more than one part of the plant. Cinnamon essential oil, for example, may come from the bark, leaves, or roots of the cinnamon tree. However, the essential oil comprises only a small portion of a plant, usually about 1 to 2 percent. To make one pound of ylang-ylang essential oil, for example, requires fifty pounds of flowers. Eight million jasmine flowers are needed to produce a kilo of jasmine essential oil.

Aromatherapists make a distinction between essential oils and carrier oils. Carrier oils—also called base oils, vegetable oils, or fixed oils—do not evaporate as fast as or have the pungent odor of essential oils. A carrier oil is blended with essential oils in order to dilute the essential oils and speed their delivery. Common carrier oils include apricot, avocado, grapeseed, jojoba, and almond oil.

PSYCHOLOGY OF SCENT

Fragrances can have a powerful effect on the mind because olfactory stimuli are more commanding than visual or aural stimuli. For better or worse, certain odors have an immediate and abrupt effect on the mind, triggering vivid memories and bringing about sudden changes in mood. As a measure of how potent odors can be, consider the fact that people often change facial expressions when they encounter certain smells. Neither sights nor sounds have as marked an effect on people's facial expressions or on their psychology in general.

Perhaps the most famous evocation of an odor can be found in Marcel Proust's *Remembrance of Things Past*. In this early passage from the novel, the narrator explains how the odor and taste of a madeleine, a small cake, made him recall a portion of his childhood in vivid detail:

> I raised to my lips a spoonful of the tea in which I had soaked a morsel of the cake. No sooner had the warm liquid mixed with the crumbs touched my palate than a shudder ran through my whole body, and I stopped, intent upon the extraordinary thing that was happening to me. An exquisite pleasure had invaded my senses . . . . with no suggestion of its origin . . . suddenly the memory revealed itself. The taste was of a little piece of madeleine which on Sunday mornings . . . my Aunt Leonie used to give me, dipping it first in her own cup of tea . . . . Immediately the old gray house on the street, where her room was, rose up like a stage set . . . and the entire town, with its people and houses, gardens, church, and surroundings, taking shape and solidity, sprang into being from my cup of tea . . . . When nothing else subsists from the past, after the people are dead, after the things are broken and scattered . . . the smell and taste of things remain poised a long time, like souls . . . bearing resiliently, on tiny and almost impalpable drops of their essence, the immense edifice of memory.

Some aromatherapists refer to "the psychology of scent" to explain why their healing methods work, and to some degree aromatherapy is, in fact, an attempt to manipulate people's psychology. Using essential oils, the most odiferous parts of plants, the aromatherapist seeks to elicit a deep-seated, emotional, healing response on the part of the patient. The challenge with this approach, however, is that fragrances can affect people in different ways. As John Steele, author of an article in *Aromatherapy Quarterly* titled "Brain Research and Essential Oils," put it, "In fragrance, there are no absolutes." Although people agree that some fragrances are gratifying and others are disagreeable, the individual's reaction to a fragrance is idiosyncratic and conditioned by biological, cultural, and personal factors. In other words, a rose by any other name smells sweet, but it smells sweeter to people whose olfactory nerves are more receptive; it represents different things to people who live in different cultures; and its fragrance always has personal associations for whoever is inhaling its bouquet. A skilled aromatherapist, like a skilled physician, knows the patient well and can tailor a therapeutic blend of essential oils especially suited to him or her.

Our smelling function is carried out by a thin layer of cells called the olfactory epithelium, located in the nasal cavity. Five to six million receptor cells are found in the average human epithelium (by contrast, a rabbit has 100 million receptors and a dog 220 million). Cilia, the tiny nerve fibers found at the end of olfactory receptor cells, are extremely sensitive and can detect odors in quantities of a few parts per trillion—an amount equivalent to about 0.000000000003 percent. Olfactory nerves, for example, can detect vanillin, the chemical responsible for vanilla's distinctive odor, at concentrations as low as .00000000762 grains per cubic inch.

Whereas touch, sight, and hearing are mediated by the cerebral cortex, the part of the brain responsible for reasoning and intellect, the olfactory nerves pass impulses directly to the limbic system, the prefrontal part of the brain where emotions are formed and memories are stored. Animals that depend upon their sense of smell for survival have highly developed limbic systems. The limbic system is the primitive part of the human brain that remains from the period of evolutionary history when, like the animals, we too depended on our sense of smell for survival. The close relationship between the olfactory nerves and the brain's limbic system explains why aromas can produce such startling, powerful responses— mnemonic, emotional, and instinctual—that may defy logic. Such responses are usually immediate and sudden, springing from the depths of the human psyche.

Aromatherapist Susanne Fischer-Rizzi writes about the limbic system:

Odor stimuli in the limbic system or olfactory brain release neurotransmitters—among them enkephalins, endorphins, serotonin, and noradrenaline. Enkephalins reduce pain, produce pleasant euphoric sensations, and create a feeling of well being. Endorphins also reduce pain, stimulate sexual feelings, and produce a sense of well being. Serotonin helps relax and calm, and noradrenaline acts as a stimulant that helps keep you awake. Within the limbic system resides the regulatory mechanism of our highly explosive inner life, the secret core of our being. Here is the seat of our sexuality, the impulses of attraction and aversion, our motivation and our moods, our memory and creativity, as well as our autonomic nervous system.

Recently, some psychotherapists have begun incorporating essential oils into their practice as a way of encouraging patients to explore the inner recesses of the psyche. The aromas of essential oils evoke deep emotional responses, sometimes soothing or stress-relieving and sometimes exhilarating. Similarly, massage therapists who are also skilled in aromatherapy use essential oil blends as a massage oil, combining the healing effects of touch and aroma.

A FRAGRANT HISTORY OF SCENTS AND PERFUMES

Perfumes and scents have served myriad purposes in the history of humankind. Spices were burned in the ancient temples of the Middle East as incense, and perfumes adorned kings and queens across the ancient world. The spices from which fragrances are made were so popular that wars and great expeditions were undertaken on their account. Columbus, you could say, went west on a shopping expedition for the high-grade perfumes of the East. The history of scents and perfumes demonstrates that aromatherapy is as old as medicine itself.

Perfumes in the Ancient World

The word *perfume* comes from the Latin *per fumen,* which means "to smoke." In the Egypt of the pharaohs, the word for perfume translated as "fragrance of the gods." Long before spices were blended into perfumes, they were burned as incense in religious rituals. In the ancient temples of Mesopotamia and Babylon, devotees of Enlil and Marduk had their senses awakened by the smoke of myrrh and cedarwood. The first perfume makers were undoubtedly priests. Thoth himself is supposed to have handed the recipes for making perfumes to the priests of ancient Egypt. Archeologists have discovered hundreds of alabaster perfume jars in the tombs of the pharaohs, and in some jars they could still detect a hint of frankincense.

The perfumes of the ancient world were a greasy blend of essential oils, vegetable oils, animal fat, gums, and resins. They resembled unguents more than perfumes. An Egyptian papyrus dating to 1500 B.C.E. portrays dancers with packages of unguents affixed to their heads, the sticky oil melting over their hair, shoulders, and limbs.

The Greek philosopher Socrates disapproved of perfume because it masked the distinction between sweaty slaves and their sweet-smelling masters. Nevertheless, hundreds of unguents—blends made from olive oil, almond oil, or linseed oil mixed with marjoram, thyme, sage, anise, and rose—could be purchased in the agora (marketplace) of Athens. Our word *aroma* comes from the Greek *arómata*, a term that described all things savory and fragrant, including spices, incense, perfumes, and aromatic medicines.

The early Romans at first had no interest in perfume, but they later acquired a taste for it in the foreign lands they conquered. The typical Roman extravagance soon found its expression in the immoderate use of perfumes, pomades, creams, face paints, and hair dyes. Eventually, the Roman *unguentarii*—the makers of unguents and perfumes—became as well respected as doctors and surgeons.

Perfumes in the Bible

The Bible provides many excellent examples of how ancient peoples used essential oils. The ancient Hebrews developed an appreciation for perfumes and essential oils during their exile in Babylon, which was, at the time, the center of the spice trade. They and the early Christians—the ones who could afford to, anyway—anointed their skin and hair with oils from spikenard, frankincense, and myrrh. They perfumed their bodies with cinnamon oil and used hyssop, galbanum, and cedarwood to fumigate their homes and purify their temples (Jerusalem's Temple of Solomon was built entirely of cedarwood). In their daily shopping, the inhabitants of the Holy Land liked to linger in front of the market stalls where essential oils were sold. Even the poor who couldn't afford the oils could savor the aromas and experience the oils' restorative properties.

Essential oils are usually evoked in the Bible to convey sumptuousness or suggest extravagance. Consider this passage from the Song of Solomon (4:13–15), in which the author uses the metaphor of a garden to describe her lover:

> Thy plants are an orchard of pomegranates, with pleasant fruits; camphire, with spikenard,
>
> Spikenard and saffron; calamus and cinnamon, with all trees of frankincense; myrrh and aloes, with all the chief spices:
>
> A fountain of gardens, a well of living waters, and streams from Lebanon.

In Jesus' time, spikenard was very costly. This aromatic oil, also called nard oil, is extracted from the fragile roots of the spikenard plant (*Nardostachys jatamansi*, also known as false valerian root). In biblical times, it was transported at great expense from the steep valleys of the Himalayas, where the spikenard plant grows, to the markets of the Levant. The oil was sealed in amber boxes, to be opened only when it was ready for use. Today, aromatherapists sometimes prescribe spikenard oil as a laxative and a balm for fevers.

Costly spikenard oil plays a role in the betrayal and crucifixion of Jesus. In the Book of Mark (14:3–10), Mary Magdalene—she would later become the patron saint of perfumers—anoints Jesus with spikenard oil, whereupon Jesus' disciples grumble at the extravagance. They complain that money spent for spikenard oil could be better spent feeding and clothing the poor. (A box of spikenard oil, according to some scholars, cost a year's wages in Jesus' time.) The disciple Judas Iscariot, indignant at seeing his master anointed with spikenard oil, betrays Jesus to the Pharisees:

> And being in Bethany in the house of Simon the leper, as he [Jesus] sat at meat, there came a woman having an alabaster box of ointment of spikenard very precious; and she brake the box, and poured it on his head.
>
> And there were some that had indignation within themselves, and said, Why was this waste of the ointment made?
>
> For it might have been sold for more than three hundred pence, and have been given to the poor. And they murmured against her.
>
> And Jesus said, Let her alone; why trouble ye her? she hath wrought a good work on me.
>
> For ye have the poor with you always, and whensoever ye will ye may do them good: but me ye have not always.
>
> She hath done what she could: she is come aforehand to anoint my body to the burying.
>
> Verily I say unto you, Wheresoever this gospel shall be preached throughout the whole world, this also that she hath done shall be spoken of for a memorial of her.
>
> And Judas Iscariot, one of the twelve, went unto the chief priests, to betray him unto them.

In Psalm 45 (7–8), the author contrives a metaphoric essential oil called "the oil of gladness." He goes on to describe the exquisite aroma of the righteous man's clothing by likening it to several essential oils:

> Thou lovest righteousness, and hatest wickedness: therefore God, thy God, hath anointed thee with the oil of gladness above thy fellows.
> All thy garments smell of myrrh, and aloes, and cassia, out of the ivory palaces, whereby they have made thee glad.

Like spikenard, myrrh was a precious commodity in biblical times, and as such, it made a suitable gift for the infant Christ. Myrrh, a resin, or dried sap, comes from the shrub *Commiphora myrrha*. Today it is used as an ingredient in incense, but in ancient times it was used as well in perfumes and oils. Egyptian women are thought to have worn pieces of cloth soaked in myrrh oil around their necks, the idea being that the heat of their bodies would activate the myrrh fragrance throughout the day. Dioscorides, Pliny, and other Greek and Roman physicians valued myrrh's antiseptic qualities and made it an ingredient in healing salves.

Frankincense is derived from the gummy resin of the frankincense tree (*Boswellia carterii*). Its name means "true incense" in medieval French. Frankincense was the most precious aromatic substance in biblical times. In the Book of Exodus (30:34), God instructs Moses to mix frankincense in the incense to be burned on the Ark of the Covenant, the first altar: "Take unto thee sweet spices, stacte, and onycha, and galbanum; these sweet spices with pure frankincense: of each shall there be a like weight."

To this day, frankincense, along with storax and benzoin, is burned in incense during Roman Catholic masses. It was to the Arabian Peninsula what petroleum is today—a valuable commodity and the chief source of income. Camel caravans carried frankincense along the Spice Trail to markets in Alexandria and Damascus, a journey of two-and-a-half months. Frankincense was also transported by ship across the Red Sea to Egypt. A glance at a map makes this voyage seem easy, but fickle trade winds on the Red Sea made it extremely hazardous, and for a time only Arabian sailors were able to complete the voyage successfully. By the first century C.E., however, Roman sailors had learned how to navigate the Red Sea, and they wrested the frankincense trade from the Arabs. As a result, Arab traders who had once been counted among the richest men in the world were reduced to being nomads.

The Age of Distillation

Perfumes disappeared in Europe after the collapse of the Roman Empire—and were rediscovered a thousand years later by the Crusaders, who, like the Romans before them, acquired a taste for them in the Holy Land. The Arabian Peninsula, meanwhile, became the center of the perfume trade, with Arab pharmacies stocking myrrh, cloves, camphor, juleps, and rose water. In the eleventh century C.E., the Arab physician Avicenna invented the process of alcohol distillation, using it to create rose water. This new process—which allowed the manufacture of perfumes without a heavy oil base—quickly gained popularity. In Arab homes, it became customary to keep bowls of rose water on hand so that family members and guests could sprinkle the water on themselves and be refreshed.

The sophisticated new perfumes—rose water, jasmine, patchouli, and others—had the effect of changing people's minds about what perfume was and what it could be. Perfume began to lose its reputation as a healing potion and became, instead, depending on your point of view, an alluring fragrance or a camouflage for offensive body odor. As well as being used on the skin, it was sprinkled onto clothing, furniture, and linen. Wealthy Europeans of the Middle Ages and Renaissance doused themselves with the fragrances of the day, and kings and queens even hired their own perfumers. Because perfumes were used so profusely in the court of Louis XV, it became known as *la cour parfumée*, or "the perfumed court."

Eventually, toilet-water blends took the place of rose water and other single-flower fragrances. The first may have been Carmelite water, a toilet water prepared by nuns of the St. Juste Carmelite abbey for Charles V of France. It consisted of lemon balm, orange flower, angelica root, and various spices. The most popular toilet water was Eau de Cologne, a mixture of lavender, bergamot, neroli, and rectified grape spirit. French troops stationed in Köln, Germany, discovered it on apothecary shelves—its official name was Aqua Admirabilis- -and gave it its French name. It became the favorite of Napoleon and did a brisk business throughout Europe in the nineteenth century.

In the twentieth century, advances in organic chemistry revolutionized the perfume industry. Instead of blending essential oils, chemists now blend molecules extracted from essential oils to create fragrances unknown in the past. Perfumers have literally thousands of synthetic fragrance materials to work with as they blend new perfumes. Fragrances have become extremely complex and alluring, and the rarified new scents mark the beginning of a new stage in the history of perfumes.

THE FOUNDERS OF AROMATHERAPY

The man credited with inventing aromatherapy was a French chemist named René-Maurice Gattefossé. In 1928, working in the laboratory of his family's perfume manufacturing plant, Gattefossé burned his hand badly in an experiment. Without thinking, he plunged his hand into the nearest vat of liquid, which happened to be lavender essential oil. To his surprise, the oil soothed his inflamed skin and soon healed it. Gattefossé then embarked on a series of experiments to test the healing powers of various essential oils. He published the results in *Aromathérapie,* an influential book that gave the new healing discipline its name.

Another Frenchman, an army surgeon named Jean Valnet, took up the practice of aromatherapy during World War II. Dr. Valnet used essential oils as antiseptics to treat the soldiers under his care. Soldiers who slept in the pine forests, he observed, had fewer respiratory infections. He concluded that the aroma of pine trees kept the soldiers healthy. Dr. Valnet made the study of essential oils his life's work. His *Aromathérapie: traitement des maladies par les essences des plantes* (*The Practice of Aromatherapy*), published in 1964, was the first book to describe the healing properties of different oils and examine their chemical composition.

Gattefossé's work was taken up in the 1950s by Austrian-born biochemist Marguerite Maury. In her book *The Secret of Life and Youth* (1961), Maury explored the psychological aspects of aromatherapy treatment. She proposed blending essential oils to meet the specific requirements of individuals and introduced the practice of delivering the oils by massage. Aromatherapy came into its own in the United States in the 1970s, when Robert Tisserand published *The Art of Aromatherapy* (1975), in which he presented a methodology for administering essential oils and made the practice more accessible.

Aromatherapy continues to evolve in many ways. On an individual level, psychologists use essential oils to help their patients relax. In a more broad approach, vaporizing oils in the central heating and air conditioning systems of skyscrapers—a practice sometimes called "environmental fragrancing"—has been used to kill germs and prevent sick building syndrome. And chiropractors, naturopaths, physical therapists, massage therapists, and a few physicians are using essential oils for therapeutic purposes in their practice.

HOW ESSENTIAL OILS ARE MADE

Most essential oils are extracted from plants by steam distillation. In this method, the plant material is placed in a still and subjected to pressurized steam. As the steam rises through the plant material, glands that hold essential oil open and release the oil. The oil rises with the steam and is siphoned off into another container, where the water cools and condenses back into liquid. Because essential oils and water don't mix, the oil forms a film on the surface of the water. The film is then decanted or skimmed off the top and collected. Four-fifths of all essential oils are produced by steam distillation.

The oldest method of extracting essential oil from plants, *enfleurage*, is still used to obtain oil from delicate flowers, such as those of jasmine, that cannot withstand heat processing. In the enfleurage method, flower petals are placed on purified animal fat or beeswax. Eventually, the fat or beeswax becomes saturated with oil from the flowers and a pomade is formed. The pomade is then dissolved in alcohol, which separates the essential oil from the fat or beeswax. Finally, the alcohol-essential oil combination is heated to evaporate the alcohol and isolate the essential oil.

Citrus oils are extracted in a cold press. In this simple method, the rinds are squeezed by a machine to extract the essential oil.

A new method, and one that is producing very exciting results, is carbon dioxide extraction. In this process, plant material is exposed to carbon dioxide gas at high pressure in a stainless-steel tank. Eventually, the carbon dioxide turns into a liquid solvent and extracts the oil from the plant material. When pressure is released, the carbon dioxide turns into a gas again. As such, it leaves no residue, so the essential oil is fresher and cleaner. Carbon dioxide extraction is expensive, however, and consequently so are the essential oils produced by this method.

Most aromatherapists refrain from using oils produced by what is known as the solvent extraction method. In this method, plant material is mixed with a chemical solvent, such as hexane, in a large metal vat. As the mixture is stirred, the plant material releases its essential oil. After several hours of stirring, the plant material is removed. The remaining mixture is heated or subjected to a centrifugal force machine to separate the solvent from the essential oil. Although this method is inexpensive compared to the others, the product is inert and not suitable for aromatherapy.

Top Notes, Middle Notes, Base Notes

In the nineteenth century, a perfumer named Charles Piesse invented a fragrance classification system in which each fragrance was matched to a musical note, and a successful perfume was one in which the fragrances blended into a harmonious chord. Piesse's system did not catch on, but another perfumer named William Poucher used it as a starting point to create a classification system that has been adopted by perfumers and aromatherapists. Poucher proposed that fragrances be classified in three categories: top notes, middles notes, and base notes.

- **Top notes** form the first impression. Top notes are the most volatile ingredients and are light, airy, subtle, and fleeting. Typical top notes are lemongrass and bergamot.

- **Middle notes**, also called heart notes, are the soul of the fragrance. Florals such as geranium and rose are usually chosen for the middle note.

- **Base notes** linger. Deep, tenacious oils such as patchouli or musk are selected for the base note.

Chemotypes and Quality

A chemotype (also called a chemovar) is a chemical variation that materializes in a plant subject to the soil, climate, geographical conditions, and weather where the plant grows. Plants of the same botanical species can exhibit wildly different chemical compositions, or chemotypes. Sweet basil (*Ocimum basilicum*), for example, is notorious for its chemotypes. Depending on where it is grown and how it is cultivated, the plant produces differing amounts of methyl-chavicol, linalool, and cineol. Chemotypes are extremely important to those interested in a plant's essential oils, because the chemicals found in an essential oil, of course, determine its therapeutic qualities.

On account of chemotypes, knowing the botanical species from which an essential oil was made doesn't really tell you the oil's chemical composition. To know that, you must either rely on the supplier to tell you or conduct a chemical analysis on your own. Dependable suppliers can provide a list of the chemical constituents in their essential oils. If the oil is made from a plant that is known for exhibiting different chemotypes, dependable suppliers list the chemotype as well as the botanical name of the plant. The suppliers listed in Appendix A are known to be dependable and follow these practices.

The good news regarding the chemical makeup of essential oils is that determining which chemicals are found in plants is getting easier thanks to advances in gas-liquid chromatography and infrared spectrometry. In gas chromatography, scientists place a substance in an extremely low vacuum and blast it apart into fragments. Then, similar to forensic experts piecing together the debris of a bomb blast, the scientists look at the molecular fragments and reassemble them to find out how they were put together before the blast. In infrared spectrometry, infrared radiation is passed through a sample and recordings are made on an infrared spectrum to see where the light is absorbed. By comparing the spectrum of the sample to the spectrum of known standards of identification, scientists can learn the chemical composition of the sample. Scientists can use these advanced techniques to quickly, accurately, and relatively inexpensively test the compounds in essential oils. They can find out what these compounds are with a degree of certainty never before achieved.

SHOPPING FOR ESSENTIAL OILS

When shopping for essential oils, "buyer beware" is the standard rule. Ninety-eight percent of essential oils are produced for the cosmetic and food-manufacturing industries. These oils are not of therapeutic grade. Moreover, some suppliers dilute their oils with inferior blends to cut production costs. The only way to be certain you are getting a high-grade essential oil is to purchase it from a reputable supplier. We can vouch for the suppliers listed in Appendix A. Their products are made from plants that are grown organically and processed according to the high standards of aromatherapy.

Here are a few tips for selecting high-quality essential oils:

• Purchase oil in dark glass bottles. The dark glass protects the oil from ultraviolet light, which deteriorates the oil.

- Make sure the bottles are sealed tightly. The shelf life of an essential oil is about one year. Oils lose their freshness when they are exposed to air.

- Look for a botanical name as well as an English name on the label. Suppliers should know precisely from which plant or plants their oils are made.

Playing It Safe

In order to use essential oils safely, it's important to follow a few rules:

- Do not swallow essential oils. The oils are highly concentrated and can harm the digestive tract. If you accidentally swallow an essential oil, drink as much water as you can and seek medical attention immediately.

- Always mix essential oils with a carrier oil when applying them to the skin. Due to the oils' high concentration, they can irritate and inflame the skin if applied in their pure form.

- Keep essential oils well out of the reach of children.

- If you are pregnant or nursing, do not use essential oils except under the direction of a qualified aromatherapist or doctor.

- Before using an essential oil, perform a skin test to see if you are sensitive to it. Mix a drop of the oil in question with a few drops of a carrier oil such as avocado or almond oil. Then rub the oil on the inside of your elbow and cover it with a Band-Aid for a day or two. If no reaction appears on your skin, all is well—you can safely use the essential oil.

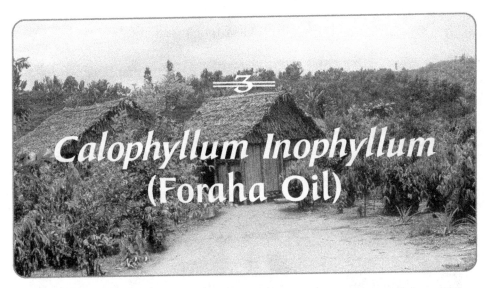

Calophyllum Inophyllum (Foraha Oil)

Wherever the *Calophyllum inophyllum* tree grows, oil from the seeds of the tree is used as a folk remedy. The tree can be found on the east coast of Africa and in Madagascar, India, Southeast Asia, the Polynesian Islands, and the Hawaiian Islands. Among folk healers, the seed oil is used to treat almost every type of skin ailment—cuts, cold sores, rashes, blisters, burns, psoriasis, acne, eczema, and even chapped lips. Polynesian women use it as a cosmetic moisturizer. In Madagascar, it is used to treat insect bites and stings. In the South Pacific and Africa, it was a traditional remedy for leprosy.

The dark green opalescent oil, known as foraha oil in Madagascar, has a pleasant, understated, slightly vegetable aroma. Malagasy foraha oil is rich and luxuriant, yet it is readily absorbed in the skin and doesn't leave a residue. It soothes, softens, and protects the skin, leaving it feeling supple and soft, and is especially helpful against sunburn. European cosmetics manufacturers have used it as an emollient in their skin moisturizers for years. *Calophyllum inophyllum* oil is so understated that it is sometimes used as a carrier oil.

In recent decades, modern medicine has discovered the benefits of *Calophyllum inophyllum*. Some of the oil's chemical compounds appear to accelerate the healing of wounds and the growth of new skin; others may be useful against HIV, the virus that causes AIDS.

INTRODUCING *CALOPHYLLUM INOPHYLLUM*

The slow-growing *Calophyllum inophyllum* tree favors sandy shores and lowland coastal forests. It grows in abundance on the humid eastern coast

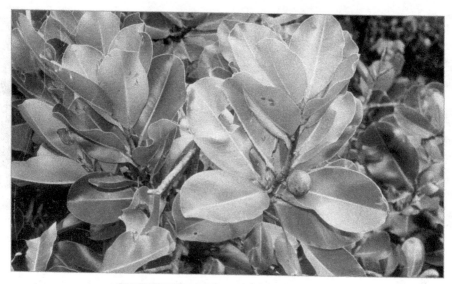

CALOPHYLLUM INOPHYLLUM (FORAHA OIL)

of Madagascar. A mature tree whose growth is not stunted by saltwater and wind can reach 60 feet (about 20 meters). The tree has spreading limbs and produces a white flower with a sweet fragrance. From July or August through November, the tree bears a bright green fruit about the size of an apricot. Inside this fruit is a spherical nut, and inside the nut is the yellow seed kernel from which *Calophyllum inophyllum* oil is made.

The fruit of the tree falls to the sand in December. After the fruit is collected, the nutlike seeds are extracted from the fruit and put out to dry and ferment on racks for one to two months. They must not be exposed to rain or humidity during this crucial time. The seeds lose a third of their weight during the drying-fermentation period. As they slowly ferment, the yellow seeds wrinkle and turn a deep brown color. The seeds become sticky with foraha oil. Finally, smelling strongly of *Calophyllum inophyllum*, the seeds are placed in a screw press and their oil is extracted.

Calophyllum inophyllum has uses above and beyond producing essential oil. Hardwood from the tree is used for building boats, houses, and furniture. And because its roots help hold sand dunes in place, the tree plays an important ecological role in maintaining healthy beaches. It often grows on the crest of a beach, where the sand dunes start. Sand dunes act as a buffer against ocean damage and flooding. They keep the beach from eroding and provide new sand for the beach after a heavy storm or strong surf has washed sand away. The roots of *Calophyllum inophyllum* are capable of penetrating many layers of sand, and the tree can withstand long periods of exposure to saltwater and violent wind. While sand dunes keep the beach from washing away, beach calophyllum keeps the sand dunes from eroding. For this reason, the trees are protected in some parts of Madagascar.

Calophyllum inophyllum was considered a sacred tree in ancient Tahiti. The Tahitians used its wood to carve tikis, their sacred objects of religious devotion. Entire forests of *Calophyllum inophyllum* grew on Tahiti previous to the arrival of Christian missionaries. When the tree lost its sacred status, those forests were cut down for timber. Now Tahitian producers of tamanu oil must gather fruit from isolated specimens of the tree. Controlled production of essential oil from *Calophyllum inophyllum* in Tahiti is not as sophisticated as it is in Madagascar.

In North America, *Calophyllum inophyllum* is cultivated as an ornamental for its glossy leaves and fragrant white flowers. Landscapers like the tree for another reason: The windblown limbs sometimes assume crooked, picturesque shapes. Because the tree is sturdy, it is sometimes used as a wayside tree. Urban landscape gardeners employ it as a windbreak for parks, parking lots, tennis courts, and other places that need shielding from the wind. However, the seeds are somewhat poisonous before they are dried, so the tree's suitability for urban locations must be considered carefully.

THE MANY NAMES OF *CALOPHYLLUM INOPHYLLUM*

Calophyllum inophyllum's botanical name comes from the Greek *kalos,* which means "beautiful," and *phullon,* which means "leaf." It has many common names. In English, the tree is known as beauty leaf (a translation of its Greek botanical name), Indian laurel (because it is supposed to have originated in India), Alexandrian laurel, and beach calophyllum (because the tree often grows on the crest of the beach).

In Tahiti, the tree is called the *ati* and its fruit is called *tamanu.* Next time you are sailing for pleasure in the South Seas and you want to locate the tree, ask for the *fetau* in Samoa, the *damanu* in the Fiji Islands, and the *te itai* in the Kiribati Islands. The tree is called *nyamplung* in Indonesia, *penaga laut* in Malaysia, and *puna* in the Lakshadweep Islands. In Hawaii it is called the *kamani* tree (sometimes spelled *kamanu*). In Madagascar, *Calophyllum inophyllum* is known as the *foraha* tree.

Because oil from the seeds of *Calophyllum inophyllum* is used in so many different cultures, it is marketed under many different names. The most common name is tamanu oil, taken from the Tahitian name for the fruit. However, the oil is sometimes called by its Malagasy name, foraha oil. In rare cases, the oil is called dilo oil, a name sometimes used in Hawaii.

When you purchase the oil, be sure to ask for the source. Enriched cocoa butter is sometimes passed off as oil from *Calophyllum inophyllum* and should be avoided. Aromatherapists favor oil from Tahiti and Madagascar. The oil from these islands is purer and more aromatic.

TRAVELS WITH *CALOPHYLLUM INOPHYLLUM*

The *Calophyllum inophyllum* tree is believed to have originated in India or Southeast Asia. From there, it spread to the subtropics of Asia, Polynesia, and the east coast of Africa.

The reddish-brown hardwood from the trunk of the tree is used in the South Seas to build outrigger canoes. The Polynesian settlers of Hawaii, arguably the most skillful sailors who ever put to sea, would have considered the tree indispensable for boatbuilding, and they brought its seeds north of the equator to Hawaii on their long journey from Tahiti, circa 400–700 C.E.

How *Calophyllum inophyllum* got from place to place south of the equator, however, is another story. *Calophyllum inophyllum* fruit has a thick, protective shell and internal air cavities that make it buoyant. It can float at sea for long periods of time without becoming waterlogged and sinking. Many thousands of years ago, seeds from *Calophyllum inophyllum* landed on a wave-swept beach on Madagascar's east coast, courtesy of the two major currents that roil the Indian Ocean, the South Equatorial Current and the Mozambique Current. The tide carried the seeds inland to a sandbank where there was enough moisture for them to germinate.

Only 120 plant species produce drift seeds, as they're called, that can float on the ocean for any length of time. The best-known and hardiest tropical drift seed is the coconut (*Cocos nucifera*). No tropical beach is complete without a coconut palm, as advertisers and movie directors know. The thick, fibrous husk of the coconut seed protects it from saltwater and enables it to travel long distances by sea. Starting from the Malay Peninsula, the coconut traveled by ocean current throughout the South Pacific.

According to C. Gunn et al., a coconut can drift at sea for 3,000 miles before sinking.

Naturalists in the nineteenth century carried on a vigorous debate as to why the same species of plants can be found on isolated volcanic islands thousands of miles apart. Some argued that migratory birds carried the seeds from island to island, but that didn't explain how plants with large seeds were dispersed. Some naturalists suggested that the islands had split in the distant past and floated away from each other, carrying the plants with them. Others believed that the islands were once connected by land bridges that were now sunk below view. The most famous naturalist of the day, Charles Darwin, noticed seeds floating on the ocean during his voyage on the H.M.S. _Beagle,_ and he was the first to propose that plants could colonize distant islands by dispersing their seeds over the ocean.

As he reported in his 1855 article "Does Sea-Water Kill Seeds?," Darwin undertook an experiment to see if plants could be dispersed by seeds floating on the ocean. For his experiment, he floated seeds in saltwater to see how long they would stay afloat. Ironically, however, the scientist who discovered natural selection and "the survival of the fittest" chose fragile seeds for his experiment. Instead of durable seeds like the coconut or _Calophyllum inophyllum,_ Darwin used common garden seeds—kidney beans, rhubarb, beet, and the like. His seeds sank to the bottom of the jar within a few days. Undiscouraged, Darwin declared that seeds could indeed travel from place to place by floating on the ocean. Instead of floating in their hulls, however, Darwin proposed that the seeds were carried in "whole or newly whole plants" and were swept to sea and deposited on a hospitable shore. He wrote:

> It should be borne in mind how beautifully pods, capsules, etc., and even the fully expanded heads of the Compositae close when wetted, as if for the very purpose of carrying the seed safe to land. When landed high up by the tides and waves, and perhaps driven a little inland by the first inshore gale, the pods, etc., will dry, and opening will shed their seed; and these will then be ready for all the many means of dispersal by which Nature sows her broad fields, and which have excited the admiration of every observer. But when the seed is sown in its new home then, as I believe, comes the ordeal; will the old occupants in the great struggle for life allow the new and solitary immigrant room and sustenance?

Besides ocean currents, seeds are dispersed in marine sea grasses, in garbage from ships, and on vegetation rafts, the large clumps of land that are sporadically set adrift by flooding and powerful ocean waves. Birds, however, are the chief means of seed dispersal. Seeds are carried in the gizzards of migrating birds and in the mud on their feet. Some seeds have sticky secretions or mechanical hooks that attach to the plumage of birds. Most seeds are capable of surviving a trip through animals' digestive systems. Thriving tomato colonies, for example, can be found in many sewage treatment plants.

MEDICINAL USES FOR *CALOPHYLLUM INOPHYLLUM*

For centuries, traditional healers have used *Calophyllum inophyllum* to treat skin ailments, arthritis, and sciatica. The leaves are heated over a fire to make them soft and then applied to cuts, boils, and sores. The oil came to the attention of the world in the 1920s when missionaries at the Makogai leprosarium in Fiji noticed patients applying dark green oil to the lesions on their skin. The oil turned out to be *Calophyllum inophyllum* (the Fijians called it dolno oil; *dolno* means "no pain" in their language). A sister at the leprosarium, Sister Marie-Suzanne of the Society of Mary, undertook her own experiments and discovered that the dark green oil was indeed useful in relieving neuritis, the painful swelling of the peripheral nerves that sometimes accompanies leprosy. She developed an ethyl-ether injection from the oil that was used to treat neuritis as well as sciatica and shingles.

After its success in treating neuritis was proved, oil from *Calophyllum inophyllum* was shipped to France and investigated for its antineuralgic properties. Soon after, however, French researchers hit on another, more valuable use for the essential oil—as a salve for damaged skin. French medical literature of the 1930s reports many cases in which the oil was used successfully to treat wounds, burns, and cuts. In one famous case, a woman with a gangrenous ulcer on her leg was admitted to St. Louis Hospital in Paris. Instead of amputating her leg, the doctors decided to dress it in *Calophyllum inophyllum* oil. The ulcer healed completely.

Oil from *Calophyllum inophyllum* has anti-inflammatory and antibacterial agents. It promotes cicatrization, the "closing" of a wound due to growth of healthy tissue. But researchers aren't sure how the oil accomplishes its magic. Following are reports of some clinical trials and studies that were undertaken on *Calophyllum inophyllum*.

Calophyllum Inophyllum and HIV

The seeds of *Calophyllum inophyllum* are known to contain coumarin. This interesting substance is the chief ingredient in Coumadin, the anticoagulant drug. The coumarin in *Calophyllum inophyllum* and other plants hinders the liver's production of vitamin K, the vitamin that makes blood clot so that wounds stop hemorrhaging. People who have had strokes often take Coumadin to keep blood clots from forming and new strokes from occurring. Coumarin is also the chief ingredient in the rat poison Warfarin. This poison interferes with the rats' vitamin K production and causes them to bleed to death.

The coumarin in *Calophyllum inophyllum* contains two compounds—calanolide A and calanolide B—that may be useful against HIV, the human immunodeficiency virus that causes AIDS. In vitro studies have shown that calanolide A and B molecules inhibit the HIV virus. They do so by attaching themselves to an enzyme that the virus needs to reproduce, thereby disabling the virus's reproduction. In 1998, researchers at the Université de Sherbrooke in Québec analyzed the calanolide molecules in *Calophyllum inophyllum* and discovered significant amounts of calanolide B. Experiments are currently underway on this compound, and if it proves useful against HIV, *Calophyllum inophyllum* may become a practical source of calanolide B.

By the way, the discovery of calanolide A and B represents a milestone. Starting in 1987, researchers from the University of Illinois in Chicago, working on behalf of the United States National Cancer Institute, combed the jungles of Sarawak state in Malaysia for plants they hoped to develop into anticancer drugs. Local healers pointed them to the bintangor tree, a sister tree to *Calophyllum inophyllum* whose scientific name is *Calophyllum lanigerum*. Calanolide A and B were first isolated from the seeds of this tree. After the compounds' anti-HIV properties were discovered, the government of Sarawak province entered into a contract with an American company called MediChem Research to develop and commercialize drugs from the compounds. Historically, plant explorers and the companies they work for have not shared the profits of their discoveries with foreign peoples or governments. In this case, however, the government of Sarawak state is putting up half of the money needed for the research. In return, it will receive half of the profits of drugs commercialized from calanolide A and B. Scientists from Malaysia, meanwhile, have been invited to work and study at the MediChem Research labs in the United States.

The discovery of calanolide A and B also represents a cautionary tale. When botanists returned to Sarawak state in 1993 to obtain more seed samples from the bintangor tree from which the original samples were collected, they found only a tree stump. The tree had been cut down for firewood. Even worse, seeds taken from nearby bintangor trees did not contain the same calanolide A and B molecules. These molecules had to be synthesized in the laboratory from the original samples. The moral: Our health depends on preserving the biodiversity of plants and animals.

Calophyllum Inophyllum and Cancer

Scientists at Meijo University in Japan were also interested in the healing properties of coumarins from *Calophyllum inophyllum*. In this instance, however, they isolated ten 4-phenylcoumarins from *Calophyllum inophyllum* with an eye toward seeing whether the compounds would inhibit the Epstein-Barr virus in the test tube. All ten compounds showed inhibitory activity. However, one compound in particular, calocoumarin-A, showed special promise. The scientists tested it in vivo on skin tumors in laboratory mice. The compound "exhibited a marked inhibitory effect" on the tumors. This experiment shows that compounds in *Calophyllum inophyllum* may be effective in treating cancer.

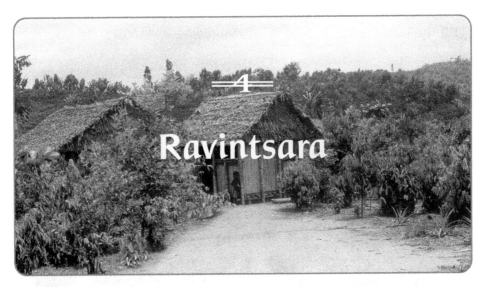

Ravintsara

*R*avintsara means "good leaf" in Malagasy (*ravint* means "leaf" and *sara* means "good for you"). The leaf of the tree is used in the central highlands of Madagascar as a folk remedy. Tea made with the leaves is used to treat stomachaches and headaches. People who have colds and bronchial ailments rub ravintsara oil onto their chests and throats and steam the leaves and inhale the vapors. The leaves are also used as condiments in certain culinary specialties. Malagasies have given the tree "noble" status on account of its aesthetic and therapeutic virtues. Ravintsara trees were planted on the estates of the noble families of Madagascar, and they can be found in many yards in the highlands. When the French colonists noticed how the Malagasies revered the ravintsara leaf, they planted ravintsara trees on the grounds of hospitals and missions so they, too, could take advantage of its medicinal benefits.

The last decade has witnessed a surge of interest in ravintsara oil as aromatherapists and herbal healers have discovered its therapeutic properties. Unfortunately, ravintsara oil is often hard to come by. Very little controlled cultivation of the oil is conducted in Madagascar. Producers of ravintsara oil have to obtain the leaves where they can. Usually that means roaming towns and villages and buying leaves from whoever will sell them. A few producers, including Phael-Flor, are planting and cultivating the trees for mass production of ravintsara oil, but we will have to wait a few years for the trees to mature and production methods to be established.

INTRODUCING RAVINTSARA OIL

Ravintsara oil is extracted from the leaf of the tree by steam distillation.

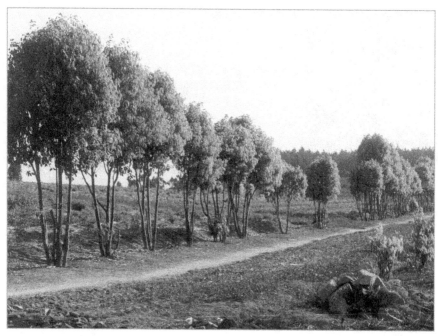

RAVINTSARA

It is limpid and colorless and has a deep, camphorous, woody, slightly floral scent. Although it smells camphorous, the oil contains no camphor. Its rich supply of cineol (comprising 50 to 70 percent of the oil) is responsible for the camphorous aroma.

The oil is soothing and relaxing, and it is popular in massage oil blends. Aromatherapists believe that the oil can travel deep into muscle tissues and joints. Some have suggested that the oil has antiviral properties, and it is thought to relieve rheumatism and joint inflammation.

THE RAVINTSARA TREE—ANOTHER FALSE CAMPHOR?

The ravintsara tree grows to 15 feet (5 meters) in height. It is grown as an ornamental in the central highlands of Madagascar and thrives in the wild in the central east (Anjiro and Moramanga) and the south (Ambositra and Ambohimasoa).

In some botanical literature, the ravintsara tree is identified as *Cinnamomum camphora* J. Presl, also known as the camphor laurel. However, this classification may be in error. The camphor laurel originated in Japan and China; it now grows in many countries. Rasoanaivo, et al. have reported that *Cinnamomum camphora* was introduced to Madagascar in the mid-nineteenth century. However, leaves from the ravintsara tree are a household medicine and have been part of Malagasy culture for centuries.

Producers of essential oil from the ravintsara leaf point out that their essential oil is superior to ho wood essential oil, which is made from *Cinnamomum camphora* in China, Japan, and Sri Lanka. They argue that the ravintsara tree is, instead, a cousin of *Cinnamomum camphora*. The climate, soil composition, and natural environment of Madagascar, as extraordinary as they are, could not by themselves raise the quality of essential oil from *Cinnamomum camphora* such that it is the equal of ravintsara leaf oil.

Because the ravintsara leaf has been a folk medicine in Madagascar for so long, and because oil from the leaf is superior to oil made from *Cinnamomum camphora*, many Malagasies maintain that the ravintsara tree and *Cinnamomum camphora* are not the same tree. Some Malagasies are convinced that the ravintsara tree is yet another tree species endemic to their island. The issue is currently under study.

THE RAVINTSARA AND RAVENSARA DILEMMA

Compounding the problematic issue of the ravintsara tree's genealogy is another dilemma: Oil made from the leaf of the ravintsara tree is sometimes confused with essential oil made from a different Malagasy tree whose scientific name is *Ravensara aromatica*, Sonnerat. *Ravensara aromatica* oil is sometimes sold as ravintsara oil. Likewise, ravintsara oil is sometimes sold under the name *Ravensara aromatica*. There is an enormous amount of confusion among producers regarding these two essential oils.

Ravensara aromatica is endemic to Madagascar. Common names of the tree are ravensare, havozo, and hazomanitra. Essential oil made from its bark is called havozo (sometimes spelled avozo) oil. A few years ago, environmentalists noticed that *Ravensara aromatica* trees were being cut down for their bark. To spare the trees, environmentalists urged aromatherapists to use oil from the trees' leaves instead of their bark. Oil from the leaves was given the name aromatic ravensare (sometimes called aromatic ravensara) to distinguish it from the bark oil. *Ravensara aromatica* and the essential oils produced from it emit a faint aniseed, or licorice-like, odor. The oils enjoy a certain popularity in the United States and Europe.

The names *ravintsara* and *ravensara* are similar—and easily confused—for good reason. *Ravensara* is a Latinization of the Malagasy word *ravintsara*, which, as we've mentioned, means "good leaf." European botanists in the nineteenth century needed a scientific name for the ravintsara tree. They took the Malagasy word *ravintsara* and fashioned it into a Latin-sounding word, *ravensara*. They named the ravintsara tree *Ravensara aromatica*. In other words, the name by which we know the licorice-smelling tree today referred in the nineteenth century to the ravintsara tree. The licorice-smelling tree, meanwhile, was called *Ravensara anisata* for its aniseed odor.

One problem with naming the ravintsara tree *Ravensara aromatica* is its general lack of aroma. The ravintsara tree has a mild camphor odor, not the pungent odor of truly aromatic trees. Over time, the name *Ravensara aromatica* came to be associated with the licorice-smelling tree, which is more aromatic. Botanists and exporters were not very good at correctly naming *Ravensara aromatica* and *Ravensara anisata*. Several papers were written about one tree that were really about the other. Dealers in essential oils sometimes presumed that buyers wanted one kind of oil, no matter which name they asked for. Eventually, the name *Ravensara anisata* for the licorice-smelling tree was dropped in favor of *Ravensara aromatica*, and the ravintsara tree became *Cinnamomum camphora*.

The upshot of all this confusion is that if you are interested in essential oils from the Ravintsara leaf or *Ravensara aromatica*, be sure you know what you are getting:

• Ravintsara oil is made from the leaf of the ravintsara tree. Most dealers list the scientific name of the tree as *Cinnamomum camphora* (although, as this chapter points out, this designation may be incorrect). Dealers who offer oil made from the bark of the ravintsara tree are really dealing in oil from *Ravensara aromatica*.

• Essential oil made from the bark of *Ravensara aromatica* is called havozo (sometimes spelled avozo).

• Essential oil made from the leaf of *Ravensara aromatica* is called aromatic ravensare (or aromatic *ravensara*).

• So-called ho wood oil, which is made from *Cinnamomum camphora*, does not come from Madagascar. Ho wood essential oil is made from trees growing in Japan, China, and Sri Lanka. These trees share the same botanical properties as the *Cinnamomum camphora* that grows in Madagascar, but their leaves are composed mostly (in the 90 percent range) of linalool. Chinese ho wood oil, in fact, has replaced rosewood as the preferred source of natural linalool. (Ho wood oil does not come from the wood of the tree—it is made from the leaves.)

You can always rely on your nose to tell which oil you are getting. Ravintsara oil has a faint camphor odor, whereas oil from *Ravensara aromatica* smells of anise. If you know the chemical composition of the oils, take note of the cineol content. *Ravensara aromatica* in its true form has a very low cineol content, whereas leaves from the ravintsara tree have a 50 to 70 percent cineol content.

The name *raventsara* sometimes appears in papers and commercial literature about the ravintsara leaf. This word is an attempt to build a bridge between the Malagasy *ravintsara* and the Latinized *ravensara*. Anyone who deals in essential oils with the name *raventsara* probably isn't dealing with a full deck.

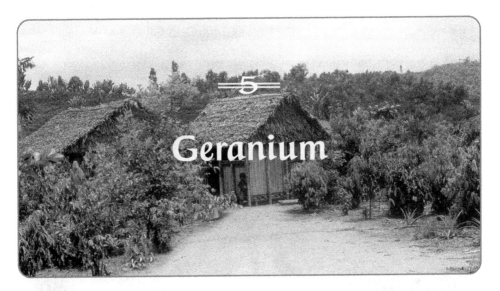

Geranium

Geranium oil is steam-distilled from the leaves, stalks, and flowers of various plants in the *Pelargonium* genus. Perfumers favor the so-called Bourbon variety, which is made from *Pelargonium roseum* grown in the central highlands of Madagascar and on Réunion Island. The Bourbon variety of geranium oil, sometimes known as the rose geranium variety, is heavy, olive green, and richer than other geranium oils. It has a rosy, slightly sweet, minty fragrance and an uplifting effect. Its rosy aroma comes from the geranoil in the leaves. This alcohol is found in higher concentrations in *Pelargonium roseum* than in other pelargoniums.

Geranium oil from *Pelargonium roseum* has a remarkable staying power and blends excellently with other oils. Cosmetics manufacturers purchase the majority of rose geranium oil for use in their creams, lotions, soaps, shampoos, and other products. Geranium oil is often used to scent soaps and detergents because it can hold its own in soap's alkaline environment. Recently, the Bourbon variety has found favor with aromatherapists. Although it is more expensive than other geranium oils, aromatherapists recognize the Bourbon variety's superior fragrance and healing power. And because it is versatile and blends well, Bourbon geranium oil offers the creative aromatherapist an opportunity to experiment with new combinations and blends.

INTRODUCING GERANIUM OIL

About 700 species of pelargoniums exist. Geranium oil is made not only from *Pelargonium roseum* but also from inferior types of pelargoniums, including *Pelargonium graveolens, Pelargonium capitatum, Pelargonium*

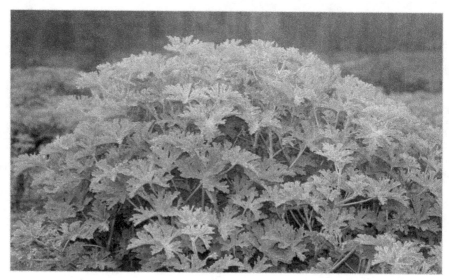

GERANIUM

asperum, and *Pelargonium odorantissimum.* These pelargoniums are cultivated for their essential oils in Madagascar, Réunion Island, Morocco, Algeria, Egypt, Uganda, and China. Although the plants are known as geraniums, they are really pelargoniums; they belong to the *Pelargonium,* not the *Geranium,* genus. (We explain this confusion shortly.)

Pelargonium roseum is called the Bourbon geranium because the plant was first cultivated on Réunion Island, formerly one of the Bourbon Islands. These islands—located in the Indian Ocean close to Madagascar— were named after the Bourbon kings of France. When the French Revolution deposed and beheaded Bourbon King Louis XVI, Réunion Island ceased to be a Bourbon island. By decree, the victorious revolutionaries named the island Réunion to commemorate a seminal event in the French Revolution: the reunion of volunteer army units from Marseilles with the National Guard for the assault on the Tuileries Palace on August 10, 1792. (The French national anthem, *The Marseillaise,* is so named on account of its popularity with those same volunteer army units from Marseilles.) Following Napoleon's downfall, the Bourbons were restored to the throne and Réunion Island briefly became a Bourbon island again. The Revolution of 1848, however, changed the island's name back to Réunion, and so it remains to this day.

Pelargonium roseum, the plant from which the Bourbon variety of geranium oil is made, is a hybrid of *Pelargonium radens* L'Her and *Pelargonium capitatum* H. E. More. The flower was brought to Madagascar in the 1920s from nearby Réunion Island. The soil composition and climate in parts of Madagascar are very similar to Réunion Island and permit *Pelargonium roseum* to be grown there. In 1925, Madagascar exported 800 kilograms of Bourbon geranium oil to France, but production soon fell into decline. In recent years it has picked up again, thanks to the high prices being paid for top-grade Bourbon geranium oil. In 1996, Madagascar exported 500 kilograms of the oil.

CARL LINNAEUS AND THE GERANIUM MISTAKE

The binomial system of naming plants and animals was established by a Swedish naturalist named Carl Linnaeus (1707–1778), the father of taxonomy. Contrary to popular belief, Linnaeus did not invent the two-name system. Gaspard Bauhin, a Swiss botanist and anatomist, introduced it in the seventeenth century. Linnaeus, however, standardized the names. For his *Species Plantarum,* a book in which he attempted to catalog all known plant and animal species, Linnaeus assigned binomials to the common names of plants and animals. In this way, he made it possible for botanists and zoologists to be certain which plants and animals they were studying. *Species Plantarum* described about 7,700 species of plants and 4,400 species of animals. By international agreement, *Species Plantarum,* 10th edition, volume 1, published in 1758, was established as the official authority for botanical and zoological names. Linnaeus's book became the starting point for referring to species of plants and animals.

In the binomial system, an animal or plant's genus name comes first, followed by its species name, an epithet that describes it. The genus name is capitalized and the species name is lowercased. *Pelargonium roseum,* for example, is in the genus *Pelargonium* and belongs to the species *roseum.* Usually, the species name refers to a shape, color, or other feature that distinguishes the plant within its genus. An authority citation—often the name of the taxonomist, botanist, or zoologist who named the species—can also be tagged on if distinguishing the animal or plant further is necessary. *Pelargonium roseum,* for example, is a hybrid of *Pelargonium radens* L'Her and *Pelargonium capitatum* H. E. More. Previous to Linnaeus's binomial naming system, plants had ridiculously long names. For example, the common carnation was called *Dianthus floribus solitari-*

is, squamis calycinis subovalis brevissimus, corollis crenatis. Linnaeus named it *Dianthus caryophyllus,* for which we should all be grateful.

Unfortunately, Linnaeus made an error when it came to geraniums. Today, what we call geraniums fall in two separate genera: *Geranium* and *Pelargonium.* In *Species Plantarum,* however, Linnaeus lumped together all plants in what are now the *Geranium* and *Pelargonium* genera in the *Geranium* genus. Although fellow naturalists such as Joannis Borman and others argued for a separate *Pelargonium* genus, Linnaeus ignored them. The mistake was corrected within a generation, when French magistrate and botanist Charles-Louis L'Héritier de Brutelle made the case for a *Pelargonium* genus. He argued that flowers of the *Pelargonium* species have irregular flowers with seven to ten fertile stamens, whereas flowers of the *Geranium* species are regular in shape and have ten fertile stamens. The new genus *Pelargonium* was born and accepted by botanists.

By this time, however, it was too late to change the common name of the genus. Pelargoniums from Africa—Zonals, Regals, Ivys, Martha Washingtons—had become popular in England and America. The African flowers were known to their loving public as "geraniums." The nurserymen who raised and sold them were loathe to change the name of the popular flower to "pelargonium," a difficult-to-pronounce name, even if it was botanically correct.

Today, gardeners make a distinction between annual geraniums (those of the genus *Pelargonium*) and hardy geraniums (those of the genus *Geranium*), but that is as far as it goes. Most geranium fanciers would not know what you were talking about if you complimented their pelargoniums.

By the way, Carl Linnaeus also devised a classification system for plants—it has since been abandoned—whereby plants were categorized according to the configuration and number of their sexual organs. He counted the number of pistils and stamens on plant buds and classified the plants accordingly. He even wrote of plant "nuptials" and referred to stamens and pistils as "husbands" and "wives." The subject being plants, some stamens had several wives and some pistils had several husbands. In his writings, Linnaeus was known to use the terminology of human love to describe plant reproduction, as in this passage from *De Systema Naturae* (1729):

> The flower's leaves . . . serve as bridal beds which the Creator has
> so gloriously arranged, adorned with such noble bed curtains, and

perfumed with so many soft scents that the bridegroom with his bride might there celebrate their nuptials with so much the greater solemnity. When now the bed is so prepared, it is time for the bridegroom to embrace his beloved bride and offer her his gifts.

Linnaeus's sexual classification system, not to mention his enticing metaphors, didn't sit well with certain prudish members of the scientific community. One of them, a Russian professor named Johann Siegesbeck, called the system "a lascivious method." He hissed, "Loathsome harlotry as several males to one female would not be permitted in the vegetable kingdom by the Creator. Who would have thought that bluebells, lilies and onions could be up to such immorality?" Linnaeus, to return the favor, named a foul-smelling little shrub *Siegesbeckia orientalis,* after the Russian professor.

In the end, Linnaeus's sexual classification system, which focused on plants' reproductive organs to the exclusion of their other morphology, proved unmanageable and was abandoned. But Linnaeus's use of binomial nomenclature and his system of hierarchical classification became the standard for botanists and zoologists.

A SHORT AND SWEET HISTORY OF PELARGONIUMS

Hybridization has made it difficult to classify the different varieties of pelargoniums. Only a few are true species; most are hybrids and mutations. About 700 varieties exist. Pelargoniums are native to the dry, arid highlands of South Africa. Their thick stems and roots enable them to store water and withstand long periods of drought. The strong scent of the leaves is distasteful to animals and protects the plants from being eaten. In its natural state, the hardy pelargonium is stunted and grows to a height of only two to three feet (0.6 to 0.9 meters). It cannot abide frosts. It is harvested when its scent is strongest, just before flowers appear. The plants are dried so that less water remains to be vaporized and the yield of oil is higher. Most of the essential oil is found in the heart-shaped, serrated leaves.

History records two stories about how pelargoniums first found their way to Europe. In one account, Europeans discovered pelargoniums in 1652 when the Dutch East India Company set up a colony in what is now Cape Town to provision ships for the East Indian trade. The Dutch settlers soon took a fancy to pelargoniums. Their governor, as the story goes, sent specimens to Holland in 1700. In the other account, botanist John Trades-cant, gardener to Charles I of England, obtained a specimen of *Pelargon-ium triste* in the early 1600s. The second account is probably the accurate one. In 1633, writing in John Gerard's *The Herball or Generall Historie of Plants* (first published in 1597), reviser Thomas Johnson described a pelargonium he saw in 1632 in the garden of John Tradescant of Lambeth.

By the start of the nineteenth century, the flower—especially the climb-ing ivy-leaf variety—became a favorite in continental Europe. Nurserymen and horticulturalists began hybridizing the species in their greenhouses. They increased the number of species to about 600. In 1786, the pelargo-nium craze spread to America, thanks to the United States ambassador to France, Thomas Jefferson, who enthusiastically dispatched pelargoniums to the John Bartram Botanical Gardens in Philadelphia.

England's early eighteenth–century infatuation with pelargoniums tapered off but revived during the Victorian period. Garden catalogs of this period offered as many as 150 varieties of pelargonium. In Victorian England, pelargoniums were a popular houseplant. They were supposed to dispel musty odors and contribute to good health. Sprigs were placed in finger bowls on the dining table so that diners could inhale the fresh scent and quicken their minds for good conversation. The Victorian obses-sion with pelargoniums lasted until World War I, when fuel for heating greenhouses was requisitioned for the war. The pelargonium stock plants could not withstand the winter cold. Cuttings for the following spring were not available because the stock plants died.

MEDICINAL USES FOR GERANIUM OIL

Geranium oil appears to regulate the flow of blood. Aromatherapists rec-ommend it for most ailments that are caused by imperfect blood circula-tion, including high blood pressure, varicose veins, hemorrhoids, and dizziness. The oil is bracing and revitalizing. Aromatherapists believe you should not take it before bed because it stimulates memory and keeps you from sleeping.

As manufacturers of skin creams know, geranium oil is also good for the skin on account of its anti-inflammatory qualities. It is often recom-mended for boils, acne, dermatitis, eczema, dry skin, and burns. It can be rubbed onto chicken pox to prevent itching and is used in healing salves that are applied to the skin after plastic surgery. It also protects the skin against aging.

The oil has a tempering quality without being a sedative. It is recommended to relieve menstrual disorders, hot flashes, premenstrual syndrome, anxiety, and stress. It is said to have antidepressant qualities and sometimes suggested as a remedy for sluggishness.

Geranium oil may be used as an insect repellent. Unlike vegetable oils, essential oils are volatile. They vaporize quickly. You can sprinkle them on clothing or linen without leaving a stain. Sprinkling geranium oil on clothing can help keep ticks, mosquitoes, and other insects at bay.

An Experiment with Geranium Oil

In 1993, a team of Russian scientists undertook an experiment to test the effects of geranium oil on skin. For their experiment, they isolated a preparation from the petals of _Pelargonium roseum_ and applied it to hamster fibroblasts. _Fibroblasts_ are the cells that make up collagen, the substance that forms the structural mesh that shapes and nurtures skin, bones, muscles, tendons, and cartilage. Fibroblasts in the skin are what make the skin soft and flexible. They play an important role in healing because they form the fibrous tissue that covers cuts and scrapes. Studying fibroblasts is the standard technique for examining the effects of radiation.

The Russian team discovered that geranium oil had "a pronounced radioprotective effect" on the fibroblasts. This experiment confirms what aromatherapists and others have known for a long time—geranium oil is good for the skin. The experiment suggests that the oil might be a viable ingredient in sunscreens and sunblocks.

OBTAINING BOURBON GERANIUM OIL

There is an enormous amount of confusion about pelargoniums, especially in the perfume sector. The genealogy of the various species is lost. We may never know which plants are the true parents of the pelargoniums used for essential oils in different parts of the world.

Before you purchase geranium oil, make sure you know what you are getting. _Pelargonium roseum_ is the plant from which Bourbon geranium oil, also known as rose geranium oil, is made. Despite the "odor" in its botanical name and despite what some distributors of essential oils claim, _Pelargonium odorantissimum_ is not the plant from which Bourbon geranium oil comes. Nor is *Pelargonium graveolens.* Oils made from these pelargoniums originate from Algeria, Morocco, and Egypt. They are not as green or as heavy as Bourbon geranium oil from Madagascar and Réunion. They do not emit the strong whiff of roses or the tang of mint. And if a producer tries to pass off oil from a plant of the *Geranium* genus as geranium oil, run like the dickens! Geranium oil comes from plants of the genus *Pelargonium.*

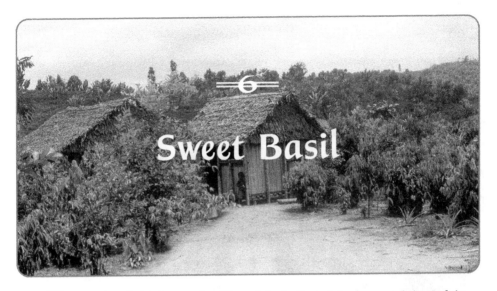

Sweet Basil

S weet basil (*Ocimum basilicum*) is believed to have originated in India or Persia. It grows in temperate and tropical climates throughout the world, including Europe, Asia, and North and South America. The word *basil* is from the Greek *basileus,* which means "king." The genus name *Ocimum* is a Latin derivation of the Greek word *ózein,* which means "to smell" (the English words "ozone" and "odor" come from this same Greek root).

Most people know sweet basil as a culinary herb used to flavor salad dressings, stews, and sauces. Food manufacturers often use basil essential oil as a flavoring (and as a way to get around having to put dried basil leaves in their products). Basil oil is also found in soaps, shampoos, and perfumes. The oil has a strong characteristic fragrance. It is sweet and spicy and is often used to construct the top note in men's colognes and toiletry products.

The oil is extracted by steam distillation from the leaves of the sweet basil plant. It falls into two categories: true sweet basil and exotic sweet basil. Oil from true sweet basil is produced in the United States and Europe. Exotic sweet basil oil, sometimes known as Réunion basil oil, comes from a handful of islands in the southwest corner of the Indian Ocean: Réunion, the Comoros, the Seychelles, and Madagascar. The exotic variety's high methyl-chavicol content gives it a faint licorice-camphor odor that is appealing to aromatherapists.

Madagascar exports approximately 400 to 600 kilograms of exotic sweet basil oil annually. The plant is cultivated in the north, around Ambanja (and formerly in the southwest in Tuléar Province). Basil oil from Mada-

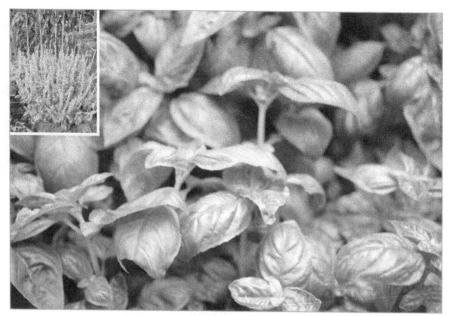

SWEET BASIL

gascar is stimulating, refreshing, purifying, and uplifting. It is pale yellow with a hint of green and has a faint licorice aroma, with balsamic undertones. It is often blended with other green-note oils, including geranium, sage, lime, and citronella.

CHEMOTYPES OF BASIL

You have to be especially careful when choosing a basil oil. Essential oils made from basil vary considerably. Several centuries of crossbreeding by horticulturalists, variability within the *basilicum* species, and the natural diversity of fragrances add up to basil oils that differ greatly from one another. Compounding this problem is the matter of chemotypes. As we discussed in Chapter 2, a chemotype is a chemical variation that appears in a plant, subject to the conditions under which it is cultivated. All plants produce chemotypes, but the variety of chemotypes in basil is extraordinary. The plant is particularly reactive to the environment in which it is cultivated.

Essential oil is found in 0.20 to 1.0 percent of the dried leaves of *Ocimum basilicum*. The major compounds of the oil are methyl-chavicol (estragole), linalool, 1,8-cineol, methyl-cinnamate, and eugenol. The exact amount of each varies considerably from species to species, and hardly any basil contains all of these chemical compounds. If you can, ask suppliers to provide a breakdown of the chemical composition of their basil oils so you know what you are getting.

Basil oil from Madagascar is high in methyl-chavicol (in the 75 to 85 percent range). This accounts for the oil's faint licorice aroma and hint of camphor. The oil is low in linalool, methyl-cinnamate, and eugenol. The chemical composition of basil oil from Madagascar indicates that it belongs to the same chemotype as basil oil from Réunion and the Comoro Islands. Basil oils from those islands are prized by some members of the aromatherapy community.

In contrast to basil oil from Madagascar, the Mediterranean basil cultivated in Europe is usually characterized by linalool and 1,8-cineol. Basil oil from India and Pakistan is high in methyl-cinnamate. Oil from Egypt and Morocco, with its clovelike odor, is high in eugenol.

A 1976 study found that methyl-chavicol (estragole) caused liver cancer in laboratory mice. Is estragole carcinogenic? Probably not, but the jury is still deliberating. The United States Food and Drug Administration (FDA) has given estragole generally recognized as safe (GRAS) status. A report by the European Commission on Health and Human Protection, however, determined that estragole is carcinogenic, although the Commission could not determine a threshold of carcinogenicity. Reducing exposure to substances that contain estragole is recommended. (In addition to basil oil, estragole is found in Mexican avocado leaf, tarragon, and fennel oils.) To confuse matters even further, a 1987 study on human subjects found that estragole poses little human risk for cancer, because humans excrete carcinogenic metabolites more readily than animals. But until more is known about estragole, it may be wise to avoid exposing children to it and to combine basil oil with other oils in aromatherapy treatments.

BASIL IN FOLKLORE

The folklore of basil is voluminous. The plant seems to inspire all kinds of myths and stories. Perhaps the spicy fragrance of basil stimulates the part of the brain that controls the imagination. At any rate, you can travel to almost any culture and find basil in the folklore.

In India, where basil was probably first cultivated, holy basil (*Ocimum sanctum*) is sacred to the Hindu god Vishnu and his avatar Krishna. Devotees of Lord Vishnu wear necklaces made from basil stems and grow holy basil on the verandas and courtyards of their homes. To inaugurate the annual marriage season, priests marry Lord Krishna to holy basil each October in a ritual ceremony called the *Tulsi Vivaha.* This ceremony commemorates a story from the *Puranas,* a collection of Indian mythology, in which Krishna's wives, to fetch Krishna from heaven, are required to present the gods with valuables equal in weight to Krishna. All the wives' jewels and riches could not tip the weighing scale, according to the story, but one wife, plucking some basil leaves from a nearby shrub, put them on the scale in place of the riches. The basil leaves by themselves tilted the scale and the gods returned Lord Krishna to his wives.

Basil was a symbol of mourning to the early Greeks. According to the folklore of the Greek Orthodox Church, the herb was found in Christ's tomb after the resurrection, and it is considered a symbol of regeneration. It is mixed in holy water and used to decorate altars. The voodoo devotees of Erzulie, the goddess of erotic love, place basil on her altar to procure favors and sympathy. Haitian shopkeepers sprinkle basil water on the street in front of their shops to bring prosperity and protect against evil. Under the name St. Joseph's wort, basil is an ingredient in witches' potions. According to traditional Italian custom, a woman places the plant on her balcony to announce that she is receiving suitors.

Ancient Greeks and Romans thought that basil caused insanity and hostility. To make the herb grow, they believed, it was necessary to curse and swear while sowing the seeds. Something of this idea has been handed down to the modern-day French, for whom "sowing basil" (*semer le basilic*) means to curse and rant. Citing the early Greeks' ideas about basil, some scholars have argued that basil got its name not from the Greek word for king, *basileus,* but from the Greek word *basiliskos,* or basilisk, the mythological king of the serpents whose mere glance is fatal.

Basil was associated with the scorpion in some cultures. This idea originated in astrology. Basil, according to ancient Greek and Roman astrologers, is ruled over by Scorpio, the zodiac sign of the scorpion. The ancient Greeks thought that scorpions bred under pots of basil. By the seventeenth century, the idea that scorpions and basil go together had died out, but French botanist Joseph Pitton de Tournefort (1656–1708) revived it in his *Institutiones Rei Herbariæ* when he included this story in his description of basil:

A certain Gentleman of Sienna, being wonderfully taken and delighted with the Smell of Basil, was wont very frequently to take the Powder of the dry Herb, and snuff it up his Nose; but in short Time, he'd turn'd mad and died; and his Head being opened by Surgeons, there was found a Nest of Scorpions in his Brain.

This chapter would not be complete if it didn't include the oddest description of basil, which comes from Nicholas Culpeper (1616–1654), author of *The English Physitian: or An Astrologo-Physical Discourse of the Vulgar Herbs of This Nation.* Culpeper was a superb quack. His book gives an excellent glimpse into seventeenth-century medicine. In Culpeper's time, astronomy and alchemy had yet to be purged from the medical sciences. Culpeper's description of "Sweet Bazil" takes into account the astrological influences of Mars and Venus. And he doesn't shy away from reporting common superstitions or strange apocryphal stories. Here, we learn that basil fertilized by horse dung breeds "venomous beasts." Culpeper also passes along the tale of the man whose head sprouted scorpions, only now the poor man is French instead of Italian:

This (basil) is the Herb which all Authors are together by the Ears about, and rail at one another like Lawyers . . . And away to Dr. Reason went I, who told me it was an Herb of Mars, and under the Scorpion, and perhaps therfore called Basilicon, and then no mervail if it carry a kind of virulent quality with it: Being applied to the place bitten by a venemous Beast, or stung by a Wasp or Hornet, it speedily draws the Poyson to it; Every like draws his like. Myzaldus affirms, That it being laid to rot in Horsdung it wil breed Venemous Beasts. And Hollerius a French Physitian affirms upon his own knowledg, That an acquaintance of his by common smelling to it, had a Scorpion bred in his Brain. Somthing is the matter this Herb and Rue wil not grow together, no nor near one another: And we know Rue is as great an enemy to Poyson as any grows. To conclude: It expelleth both Birth, and After-birth; and as it helps the deficiency of Venus in one kind, so it spoils al her actions in another. I dare write no more of it.

BASIL AS A FOLK MEDICINE

The Malagasies mix powdered basil with lard and use the mixture to treat gout and rheumatism. In the Arab world, basil is supposed to ease menstrual cramps (and should therefore not be served to men, who may think their masculinity is being impugned). Basil oil is a general tonic for coughs, chills, earaches, and skin problems in Ayurvedic medicine, the traditional medicine of India. It is also an antidote for snakebites and is used to treat acne.

In *The Herball or Generall Historie of Plants,* a compendium of the properties and folklore of plants that was published in 1597, John Gerard wrote that basil's smell was "good for the heart and for the head" and its seeds "cureth the infirmities of the heart and taketh away the sorrow which commeth with melancholy and maketh a man merry and glad."

The Caribs of Guatemala use basil as an insect repellent, as do many Indians. Sir George Birdwood, a professor of anatomy at Grant Medical College in Bombay, wrote in a 1903 letter to the *Times* of London, "When the Victoria Gardens were established in Bombay, the men employed on those works were pestered by mosquitoes. At the recommendation of the Hindu managers, the whole boundary of the gardens was planted with holy basil, on which the plague of mosquitoes was at once abated, and fever altogether disappeared from among the resident gardeners."

MEDICINAL USES FOR BASIL OIL

Not surprisingly, given the number of chemotypes and the many different cultures in which basil is found, aromatherapists have numerous opinions about the proper use of basil oil. The oil is supposed to improve mental concentration and relieve stress. It is an antidepressant that stimulates the mind and awakens the senses. It is sometimes prescribed for insomnia. Blended into a massage oil (its green odor blends well with resinous scents), it is supposed to soothe aching muscles and help relieve rheumatism. Some aromatherapists believe that the oil encourages hair growth. It is also supposed to stimulate the adrenal glands, although no scientific data has been offered to prove this assertion.

A little basil oil goes a long way. Use the oil in moderation. Children and pregnant women should not use basil oil, aromatherapists say. The oil is supposed to encourage menstruation. Some aromatherapists believe that pregnant women who use basil oil run the risk of having a miscarriage.

Experiments with Sweet Basil

One of the biggest challenges facing food manufacturers is how to keep bacterial microbes and molds from spoiling their products. The doubling time of a single microbe can be as little as twenty minutes. A single microbe, therefore, can soon produce an army of bacterial microbes. Along with molds, these microbes spoil food by dying or releasing by-products into the food.

One way to keep microbes in check is to destroy them with the use of heat. However, heat processing not only kills microbes but also changes the taste of food and diminishes its nutritional value. Another technique for handling microbes is to kill them with disinfectant and antimicrobial additives such as chlorine, but these chemicals spoil the flavor of and introduce toxins into food. Food manufacturers must walk a delicate line. Keeping food fresh but also making sure it is free of molds and bacteria is a difficult balancing act. Manufacturers who produce organic and so-called natural foods have an especially difficult challenge, because they are not supposed to use chemical additives in their foods.

In recent years, food manufacturers have been revisiting the idea of using seasoning agents to kill bacterial microbes. In addition to enhancing the flavor of food, seasonings preserve it. They do so by drawing water out of bacterial cells, which ruptures the cells' membranes and destroys them. Seasonings have been used to preserve food for centuries. On behalf of the food manufacturing industry, a number of experiments have been done using essential oils from plants, including basil, as antimicrobial agents. Here are three recent examples:

- Scientists from the University of Geelong in Australia tested five varieties of basil oil for their antimicrobial activity against different bacteria, molds, and yeasts. All five demonstrated antimicrobial activity, and the growth of several kinds of bacteria was completely inhibited. The scientists were encouraged by their effort and recommended further investigations into the antimicrobial effects of basil oils.

- Scientists from the Australian Food Industry Science Centre in Victoria also conducted experiments on basil essential oils to see whether they inhibit bacterial growth. They concluded in part that washing fresh lettuce with a basil essential oil is comparable in effectiveness to washing it with 125 parts per million of chlorine bleach—a conclusion that has implications for the food processing industry.

- Scientists at the University of Tennessee used several essential oils— basil, anise, celery, carrot, cardamom, coriander, oregano, parsley, and rosemary—to examine their effect on the growth of bacterial microbes. Oil from oregano completely inhibited microbe growth, while carrot oil had no effect. Basil oil, along with coriander oil, was deemed "highly inhibitory." The scientists were also enthusiastic about the use of essential oils for food processing, and they recommended further experiments.

These experiments show that essential oils from basil and other plants have a use above and beyond aromatherapy and medicine. Essential oils can supplement or be an alternative to chlorine and other conventional antimicrobial food additives. Basil certainly tastes better than chlorine. Perhaps swimming pools will someday smell of basil instead of chlorine bleach.

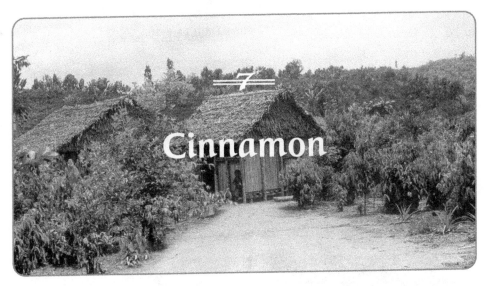

Cinnamon

Cinnamon is warming and invigorating. It seems to reach deep into the body to summon feelings of warmth and comfort. The spice and oil are made from the bark of the cinnamon tree; the oil can be made from the leaves and the roots of the tree, as well. Cinnamon oil is used in perfumes, food, soft drinks, liqueurs, and drugs.

The cinnamon produced in Madagascar comes from the bark, leaves, and roots of *Cinnamomum zeylanicum*, Blume, also known as Sri Lankan or Ceylon cinnamon (*zeylanicum* is the Latin word for Ceylon). *Cinnamomum zeylanicum* also grows in Sri Lanka, China, Sumatra, Brazil, Mauritius, India, and Jamaica.

Cinnamon oil from Madagascar is aromatic, sweet, and warm. It has a lively, animated quality and exciting overtones not found in other cinnamon. As we explain shortly, cinnamon from Madagascar is quite different from the cassia variety that is sold in the United States. True cinnamon, in fact, is hard to come by in America.

INTRODUCING CINNAMON

The cinnamon tree, an evergreen tree of the Laurel family, is native to Sri Lanka, the Malabar coast of India, and Myanmar (Burma). The bushy tropical tree requires plenty of water and warm sunlight. It prefers sandy soil and grows in elevations below 1,000 feet (300 meters). The bark is smooth and yellowish.

Cinnamon grows wild on the east coast of Madagascar in the Ambanja and Ambolotara regions and along the northwest coast between Vatomandry and Maroantsetra. Most cinnamon is collected from uncultivated

CINNAMON TREE

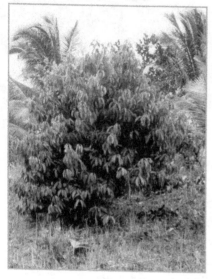

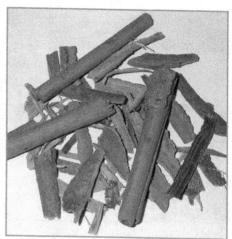

CINNAMON BARK

trees in secondary rainforests. The cinnamon tree produces a blue, juniper-tasting berry about the size of an acorn. Two birds, the rova and the marotaina, it is said, are responsible for the distribution of cinnamon trees in Madagascar. The rova and the marotaina eat the cinnamon berries and drop the seeds to the ground, where they germinate.

Cinnamon trees in Madagascar produce bark for about thirty years. Although a wild tree can grow to 30 feet (10 meters), growers coppice the tree so that the thin shoots grow close to the ground and are easy to harvest. *Coppice*—from the French *couper*, to cut—means to closely prune the top of the tree so that straight branches, or shoots, sprout from the trunk and branches. In the controlled cultivation of cinnamon, the main stem of the tree is coppiced every third year. The resulting shoots, also known as coppices, are harvested at three-year intervals for their bark.

At harvest time, the thick, scabrous bark is scraped from the coppice shoots and left to ferment in bundles for twenty-four hours. The farmers then carefully peel the corky outer layer of bark from the thin, light-colored layer underneath. Peeling requires great skill and traditionally is done in Madagascar by women laborers. The underlayer is cut into lengths called quills and left to dry for three to five days. As the quills dry, they curl and form cinnamon sticks. Cinnamon is sold in sticks or ground into a powder.

Sri Lanka is the world's leading producer of cinnamon, accounting for 11,000 to 12,000 metric tons annually. Madagascar produces about 4,000 tons of scraped and unscraped bark annually.

The word *cinnamon* came to the English language by way of the Latin *cinnamomum,* which in turn came from the Greek *kinnámoomon.* As for the Greeks, scholars disagree whether they borrowed their word for cinnamon from the Hebrew *quinamom* or the Malay *kayu manis,* which means "sweet wood."

The Chemistry of Cinnamon

Cinnamon contains 0.5 to 1 percent essential oil. The principal component and the chemical that is largely responsible for cinnamon's distinctive taste and odor is cinnamaldehyde (cinnamic aldehyde). Recent studies undertaken with gas-liquid chromatography and infrared spectrometry paint this picture of cinnamon's chemical composition:

- The bark contains cinnamaldehyde at 28 to 45 percent. How the bark is dried plays a role in the bark's chemical composition, but this subject has not been thoroughly examined by chemists or botanists.

- The leaf contains eugenol. Oil made from fresh leaves is high in eugenol. The oil from dried leaves contains benzyl benzoate.

- The root contains camphor. Although oil made from the roots of the plant smells of cinnamon, the oil is high in camphor. Some collectors supply oil from the root instead of the bark of the cinnamon tree.

Cinnamon versus Cassia

Without knowing it, many cinnamon fanciers mix cassia, not cinnamon, into their favorite desserts and pastries. In fact, the majority of ground cinnamon in the United States is actually inferior cassia. Cassia is cultivated in China. It is made from the aromatic bark of the Chinese cinnamon tree (*Cinnamomum cassia* Blume), also known as the Chinese cassia or the bastard cinnamon tree. The corky outer bark is not removed in the production of cassia. Cassia is more pungent and robust than cinnamon. It is not as delicate, sweet, or subtle as the cinnamon produced in Madagascar and Sri Lanka. The less expensive cassia is often used as a flavoring in cola drinks. It is also an ingredient in Yardley's Brown Windsor soaps.

How do you tell the difference between true cinnamon and cassia?

Unfortunately, the Food, Drug, and Cosmetic Act of 1938 permits cassia to be sold legally as cinnamon in the United States, so distinguishing between the two spices isn't a matter of reading the label on the spice jar or bottle of essential oil. Here are some tips for telling the difference between the two varieties of cinnamon:

- Cinnamon oil is a clear yellow liquid with a sweet-spicy aroma. Cassia oil is yellower and has a heavier, less refined aroma.

- True cinnamon is a tan color, whereas cassia is reddish brown to dark brown.

- Cassia bark is thicker than cinnamon bark because its outer layer isn't stripped off. For that reason, as they dry, cassia sticks curl inward from both sides toward the center. Cinnamon sticks curl from one side only and roll up like a carpet or newspaper.

- The surface of cassia bark is rough and uneven, whereas cinnamon bark is smooth.

- Because cassia bark is thicker and coarser, it cannot be ground as fine as cinnamon bark.

- Cinnamon costs about twice as much as cassia, although the cinnamon that comes from Madagascar costs less than the cinnamon from Sri Lanka, where the majority of cinnamon is grown.

- Where a distinction is made, cinnamon is used in sweet dishes that require a delicate flavor and cassia is used for spicy main dishes and curries.

If your chemistry set is handy, you can distinguish between cassia and cinnamon by taking note of how much eugenol, cinnamaldehyde, and coumarin are found in the samples. Cassia contains only trace amounts of eugenol; cinnamon is composed of 5 to 10 percent eugenol. Cassia contains coumarin; cinnamon does not. The cinnamaldehyde in cassia sometimes reaches 75 percent; the amount in cinnamon is 28 to 45 percent. Another technique for distinguishing between cinnamon and cassia is to place a drop of tincture of iodine in a fluid ounce of oil. Cassia turns dark blue; cinnamon hardly changes color.

There are two hundred or more species of cinnamon. Besides *Cinnamomum zeylanicum* and *Cinnamomum cassia*, two other species are cultivated for the commercial market: *Cinnamomum burmannii* and *Cinnamomum loureirii*. *Cinnamomum burmannii* is grown in western Sumatra, near Padang. This variety has a slightly bitter and astringent flavor. It is called Indonesian cinnamon, java cassia, fagot cassia, or Padang cinnamon. Cinnamaldehyde is the major constituent. No eugenol is found in this variety. *Cinnamomum loureirii* is grown in Vietnam and is known as Vietnamese cinnamon or Saigon cinnamon. It is similar to cassia. This variety was sold in Eastern Europe prior to the end of the Cold War. Vietnamese producers are said to be upgrading the crop to make it ready for the world market. As in cassia, cinnamaldehyde is the major constituent, at 75 percent.

A CINNAMON SUCCESS STORY IN MADAGASCAR

Cultivating cinnamon requires patience and forbearance on the part of the farmer-collector. Ideally, the bark is harvested every third year, but poor farmers have been known to strip the trees of bark without giving the bark sufficient time to grow. Sometimes the trees are pulled out of the ground so that the roots can be harvested as well as the bark. In the mid-1990s, Madagascar's cinnamon production came to a standstill due to the wanton harvesting of cinnamon bark and roots. Little cinnamon bark was left to harvest. Producers of cinnamon found themselves scouring the countryside for fresh bark. Filling a truck with the product sometimes required driving a thousand kilometers (620 miles) or more through the countryside—no easy feat on the roads of Madagascar! Finally, to give the cinnamon trees a chance to recover, the government forbade the exportation of cinnamon.

Obviously, something needed to be done to rescue the cinnamon crop. In Ambolotara, in the region of Brickaville, near the east coast and about 260 kilometers from the capital, a company called Phael-Flor decided to set up a model program for cinnamon production. Under the program, local villagers learned sustainable agricultural techniques. The idea was for villagers to make a steady, dependable income from cinnamon and for producers to have a steady supply of the crop. For its model program, Phael-Flor selected a 14-hectare (34.6-acre) site with numerous wild cinnamon trees whose growth had been stunted by bush fires. The company taught villagers how to clear competing underbrush from the deforested area in order to protect the trees from fire. It built a small production facility for steam-distilling cinnamon bark and taught villagers how to operate the facility. Instead of intermediaries trucking cinnamon to the capital for distillation, the work was done on site. This way, the villagers learned new skills and the company increased its profits.

Managers noticed the quantity of leaves left over from bark production, and they decided to distill cinnamon leaves as well as bark. Leaf production would keep the workers busy and provide income for local villagers while they waited for the cinnamon trees to mature and grow bark. Phael-Flor's decision to go into leaf production had a remarkable effect in the countryside. To make one liter of cinnamon oil requires about 100 kilos of leaves. Impoverished villagers from miles around understood that they could make money from collecting cinnamon leaves. Suddenly, villagers had a stake in preserving the forest. For miles around, villagers cleared brush from the cinnamon trees to protect them from fire.

Without realizing it, Phael-Flor had launched an extraordinary conservation effort—one with an economic incentive that will never lose its impetus as long as the distillation facility remains in Ambolotara. The fires that burn so frequently in Madagascar have stopped burning in the countryside near the Phael-Flor production facility. Local villagers, meanwhile, enjoy a higher standard of living. In recognition of its effort in preserving the environment and promoting social and economic development, Phael-Flor recently received a development grant from the U.S. Agency for International Development (USAID).

CINNAMON IN HISTORY

The prince of spices in ancient times, cinnamon was an emblem of wealth and the subject of myth and legend. The emperor Nero of Rome, perhaps feeling guilty because he had murdered his wife Poppaea, is supposed to have burned a year's supply of cinnamon at her funeral. Ancient Egyptians included cinnamon in their cosmetics and embalming formulas. The Greeks and Romans used it as a wine flavoring and an ingredient in incense. Cinnamon was also the principal ingredient in *megaleion,* the aromatic medicine that Athenians applied to wounds.

Cinnamon was sold in the marketplaces of the Levant, and the Bible mentions it several times (although the cinnamon of the Bible may well have been cassia). Says the harlot in Proverbs 7 (16–18), "I have decked my bed with coverings of tapestry, with carved works, with fine linen of

Egypt. I have perfumed my bed with myrrh, aloes, and cinnamon. Come, let us take our fill of love until the morning: let us solace ourselves with love." Love and cinnamon—who would have guessed it?

Among Arabs, especially, cinnamon was seen as an emblem of wealth. Arab merchants controlled the lucrative trade in spices throughout antiquity and well beyond the Middle Ages. Their caravans carried precious cinnamon overland from India to markets in Alexandria, Nineveh, and Babylon. To guard the secret of cinnamon's origin and to add to the spice's exotic reputation, the Arabs told wild stories about the dangers they faced gathering cinnamon in the faraway lands from which it supposedly came.

Following is an account of cinnamon's origin from the Greek historian Herodotus (484–420 B.C.E.). In Herodotus's version, cinnamon is transported to Arabia by large birds. Notice the peculiar method by which the cinnamon is acquired from the birds' nests. As you read this account, imagine the pleasure Arab merchants must have taken in telling this story to their credulous European counterparts:

> The process of collecting the cinnamon is even stranger. In what country it grows is quite unknown. The Arabians say that the dry sticks, which we call *kinnámoomon,* are brought to Arabia by large birds, which carry them to their nests, made of mud, on mountain precipices which no man can climb. The method invented to get the cinnamon sticks is this. People cut up the bodies of dead oxen into very large joints, and leave them on the ground near the nests. They then scatter, and the birds fly down and carry off the meat to their nests, which are too weak to bear the weight and fall to the ground. The men come and pick up the cinnamon. Acquired in this way, it is exported to other countries.

Four hundred years after Herodotus, the Roman historian Pliny the Elder (23–79 C.E.) mistakenly placed the origin of cinnamon in Ethiopia. At the end of this passage, he remarks on the real reason for trading—women's fashions.

> All these stories are nonsense. In fact cinnamon grows in Ethiopia, which is linked by intermarriage with the Cave dwellers. These buy it from their neighbors and bring it over vast seas on rafts which have no rudders to steer them, no oars to push them, no sails to propel them, indeed no motive power at all but man alone and his

courage. What is more, they take to sea in winter, around the solstice, which is when the east winds blow the hardest. These winds drive them on the proper course across the bays. When they have rounded the Cape, a west-north-west wind will land them in the harbor called Ocilia, so that is the trading place they prefer. They say that their traders take almost five years there and back, and that many die. On the return journey they take glassware and bronze ware, clothing, brooches, bracelets and necklaces: so here is one more trade route that exists chiefly because women follow fashion.

Cinnamon was prized in medieval Europe as a preservative and also as a staple ingredient in cooking. Meals including both meat and fruit were prepared in a single pot, and cinnamon, along with ginger, helped the flavors blend together. Over time, cinnamon became a culinary specialty rather than an ingredient in medicines.

As the centuries passed, Europeans slowly but surely pieced together the mystery of cinnamon's origins. The writings of Marco Polo, translations from Arabic writers, and reports from Christian missionaries in Asia led Europeans to believe that cinnamon grew in the Orient, probably in India or Melaka. By 1540, Portuguese mariners had found the source of cinnamon in Ceylon (now Sri Lanka) and conquered that island's Kingdom of Kotte. For the next hundred years, the Portuguese enriched themselves by monopolizing the cinnamon trade. They extracted tribute from the Sinhalese in the form of cinnamon bark and later sent their own agents into the fields to oversee the cultivation of cinnamon. To guard their monopoly, the Portuguese expelled Muslim traders from Ceylon, enslaved the Sinhalese, sank the dhows of their Arab competitors, and hanged any representatives of European countries who dared to set foot on the island.

In 1638, Dutch agents eager to capture the cinnamon trade for their country slipped into the highland Kingdom of Kandy and struck an agreement with King Rajasinha II whereby they would expel the Portuguese in return for rights to the cinnamon trade. Incidental to the agreement, Rajasinha agreed to reimburse the Dutch for military expenditures. After they defeated the Portuguese, the Dutch presented Rajasinha with such an exorbitant bill that he could not pay. In retaliation, the Dutch occupied the seaports and the richest cinnamon-producing land. The Dutch's turn at monopolizing cinnamon lasted 150 years. Like the Portuguese before them, they enslaved Sinhalese laborers and ruled the island with an iron fist. In the 1770s, desperate to meet the growing European demand for cinnamon, the Dutch introduced the controlled cultivation of cinnamon trees. This marked the first time in history that cinnamon bark was cultivated on plantations as well as gathered in the wild.

The Dutch cinnamon monopoly ended in part thanks to a courageous French botanist named Pierre Poivre (the name translates to "Peter Pepper" in English). Poivre— governor of Mauritius from 1763 to 1772—devoted himself to collecting spice plants throughout the Indian Ocean region. His goal was to break the Dutch monopoly on the spice trade and enrich the French possessions. Poivre smuggled spice plants—often at great danger to himself—to the Jardin des Pamplemousses in Mauritius. From there, the plants were distributed to French possessions in the Indian Ocean, including Madagascar. The nutmeg, clove, cinnamon trees, and pepper in the Seychelles, Réunion Island, the Comoro Islands, Mauritius, and Madagascar are descendants of plants that Poivre filched from Ceylon, the Spice Islands, and the Moluccas Islands.

By 1800, the price of cinnamon had fallen dramatically. Cinnamon trees now grew in Ceylon, Sumatra, India, the French possessions in the Indian Ocean, and even the New World. Europeans began to eat chocolate to satisfy their craving for sweets, and the popularity of cinnamon diminished. The less expensive cassia appeared in European markets to compete with cinnamon, further hurting the demand for the once-prized spice. England ruled Ceylon, the Dutch having ceded it to England at the close of the fourth Anglo-Dutch War (1780–1784). The Verenigde Oost-Indisch Compagnie—the Dutch East India Company—had gone bankrupt. The Dutch monopoly of cinnamon was broken once and for all, and cinnamon ceased to be the coveted object of ruthless traders and adventurers from Europe.

CINNAMON AS A FOLK REMEDY

Cinnamon appears as a folk remedy in many cultures. Due to its warming, comforting quality, cinnamon suggests itself as an antidote for disease. For a sore throat, says aromatherapist Jeanne Rose, place a drop or two of cinnamon oil on a sugar cube and suck. Mixed with a carrier oil and applied to the scalp, cinnamon oil is used to kill scabies and head lice. A Pennsylvania Dutch remedy for diarrhea says to stir two pinches of cinnamon into a glass of milk and drink. The Brazilian remedy for diarrhea does the Pennsylvania Dutch one better. It calls for a pinch of cloves as well as two pinches of cinnamon.

CINNAMON IN AROMATHERAPY

Aromatherapists agree that cinnamon oil is a potent substance. The oil should be taken only under the supervision of someone who understands its applications. Aromatherapists often suggest diluting it with ylang-ylang, orange, or myrrh.

The oil is believed to energize the body and increase vitality. It has an uplifting effect and relieves depression and nervous exhaustion. It is prescribed as an aid to digestion and is thought to relieve gas and bloating. Cinnamon also stimulates blood circulation in the arms and legs. Some aromatherapists suggest cinnamon oil for the relief of menstrual cramps.

MEDICINAL USES FOR CINNAMON

Many people are surprised to discover that the spice that enlivens desserts has medicinal properties, too. Cinnamon is an antimicrobial; that is, it can destroy microbes and bacteria. For example, it has been shown to inhibit the growth of *Helicobacter pylori*, the bacterium that causes stomach ulcers. It holds promise for people with diabetes, because it appears to stimulate insulin activity and thereby help the body process sugars more efficiently. Cinnamon is also a carminative and an antioxidant. It restrains the growth of fungi and yeasts and may be useful for the treatment of allergies. Following are the results of recent studies conducted to evaluate cinnamon's medicinal properties.

Cinnamon and Head Lice

Head lice (*Pediculus capitis*) are parasites that live on the scalp and neck hair of human beings, usually children who have been sharing their hats, hairbrushes, and combs with each other. The louse's six legs are ideally suited for grasping human hair. Head lice, in fact, may have evolved alongside human beings. The louse does not infest animals but dotes exclusively on humans. Females lay eggs in sacs that stick to hair. Typically, an infested person carries less than a dozen lice and as many as a hundred eggs, some unhatched and some dead. Lice feed on human blood and live about thirty days. Lice eggs are called nits. Originally, *nitpicking* meant slowly but thoroughly removing lice eggs from a person's hair.

The itching and scalp irritation that head lice cause is not nearly as alarming as the harm that comes from the well-intentioned but irresponsible use of toxic and flammable substances that eliminate lice. All head lice products contain insecticides. Malathion, lindane, and other insecticides used as pediculicides—chemical treatments to kill head lice—can bring about acute toxicity if it is used too often, especially in children, the most frequent victims of head lice. For this reason, many physicians are reluctant to prescribe pediculicides. The lice, moreover, are becoming resistant to some chemical treatments.

Because essential oils are an ingredient in many folk remedies for lice, researchers have turned their attention to essential oils as a way to treat head lice without resorting to caustic or dangerous chemicals. An August 1996 article in *Complementary Therapy Nurse Midwifery* magazine reported on a study in which the essential oils cinnamon, aniseed, red thyme, peppermint, pine, nutmeg, and rosemary in alcoholic solutions were tested in vitro against head lice. Each solution was applied, followed the next morning by a rinse comprising the essential oil, vinegar, and water. With the exception of rosemary and pine, all essential oils were deemed effective against head lice. The study noted that phenols, ketones, and 1,8-cineol were likely the chemicals that proved most toxic to the lice.

Cinnamon and Diabetes

Put simply, diabetes is the inability of the body to use glucose efficiently because of a resistance to insulin. Glucose, also known as blood sugar, comes from the carbohydrates and fat you eat. It is absorbed in the small intestine, passed through the wall of the small intestine to the bloodstream, and passed from there to the cells of the body. The cells, in turn, use glucose as energy. When there is an oversupply of glucose, as may be the case after you eat, the body stores the excess glucose as glycogen in the liver, in fat cells, and in muscle tissue. A healthy body is able to maintain a steady level of glucose in the bloodstream. It releases glycogen—that is, stored glucose—from the liver and muscle tissues when the supply of glucose in the blood falls short.

The job of insulin, a hormone produced by the pancreas, is to help glucose enter cells and to regulate blood sugar levels. Insulin helps glucose molecules pass through the wall of a cell to the interior, where it is used as energy. In people with type 2 diabetes, also known as adult-onset diabetes and non-insulin-dependent diabetes, the cells in the body become insensitive to insulin. The pancreas, therefore, has to produce more insulin to get the cells to realize that insulin is present and glucose needs to be absorbed. Because less glucose is absorbed, meanwhile, more glucose, or blood sugar, remains in the blood. Symptoms of diabetes include excessive thirst, frequent urination, fatigue, a tingling sensation in the hands and feet, and unexplained weight loss.

Ninety percent of diabetes sufferers have type 2 diabetes. In the United States, type 2 diabetes affects an estimated 16 million people, and the disease contributes to nearly 200,000 deaths annually. (Type 1 diabetes, which almost always occurs in children and young adults, is caused by a failure of the pancreas to produce insulin. Type 1 diabetics must get their insulin by injection.) Type 2 diabetes appears to be linked to obesity. Too many carbohydrates and too much fat in the diet produce excess blood sugar that can't be absorbed in the blood. Some physicians believe that glucose is not absorbed because insulin receptors on the liver, muscle, and fat cells are impaired or reduced in number. Another theory says that diabetes results when the intercellular pathways that are activated by insulin are altered.

Recently, a team of scientists from Iowa State University became interested in cinnamon after they discovered that apple pie, believe it or not, has a positive effect on blood sugar regulation. Cinnamon, of course, is an ingredient in apple pie. The researchers from Iowa determined that a chemical compound in cinnamon called methylhydroxychalcone (MHCP) was responsible. This compound, they discovered, mimics insulin and encourages the cells to recognize when glucose is present and needs to be absorbed. In other words, MHCP alerts cells to the presence of glucose. The researchers speculated that MHCP modifies cells' insulin receptors so that the cells become more alert to insulin. In a comparison of MHCP and insulin, they reported that MHCP works almost as well as insulin in triggering the chemical events by which glucose is absorbed by cells. When both MHCP and insulin were presented to cells, the total effect was greater than that observed by either substance on its own. The researchers concluded that MHCP and insulin are synergistic. For this reason, cinnamon can be very beneficial to people with diabetes. More studies need to be done on MHCP, but for now it appears that diabetics can eat dessert after all—as long as it's apple pie.

Cinnamon versus *Helicobacter pylori*

Previous to the discovery of *Helicobacter pylori* by Australian scientists Barry Marshall and Robin Warren in 1983, physicians believed that ulcers were caused by poor diet and stress. Now it appears that the bacterium *Helicobacter pylori* (*H. pylori*) is the leading cause of ulcers. This bacterium burrows into the sticky mucosal lining of the stomach to cause inflammation. Although the majority of people infected with *H. pylori* do not contract any diseases or show any symptoms, infections can cause gastritis, gastric lymphoma, stomach ulcers, and chronic duodenal ulcers (which appear in the duodenum, the first portion of the small intestine). Hypochlorhydria, a deficiency of hydrochloric acid in the stomach, may also be the consequence of a chronic *H. pylori* infection. People who suffer from hypochlorhydria cannot produce enough hydrochloric acid in their stomachs, and as a consequence, they have trouble digesting food and absorbing vitamin B_{12}.

By age sixty-five, about 60 percent of the population has been infected with *H. pylori*. How the bacterium passes from person to person is something of a mystery, but it appears that contact with infected vomit or feces may be the cause. The good news is that doctors can check for *H. pylori* with a simple blood or breath test. Infections can be treated with antibiotics. However, because getting high concentrations of antibiotics into the mucosal lining of the stomach is difficult, the antibiotic treatment can last up to four weeks and requires taking many pills.

In 1999, scientists in Israel undertook an experiment to see whether extracts of cinnamon could retard the growth of the *H. pylori* bacterium. The scientists used an ethanol and a methylene chloride extract. The cinnamon methylene chloride extract inhibited the growth of *H. pylori* at a concentration range equal to that of common antibiotics, whereas the ethanol extract counteracted the bacterium's urease activity. (Urease is an enzyme of which *H. pylori* produces large quantities.) This experiment indicates that cinnamon blocks the growth and activity of *H. pylori*, although it doesn't kill the bacterium outright.

Cinnamon as an Antioxidant

In biochemistry, molecules called antioxidants are capable to a certain extent of reversing the damage that free radicals do to body tissue. A free radical is a very unstable, highly reactive molecule with an unpaired electron. Because electrons want to occur in pairs, free radicals steal electrons from other molecules. This process is called oxidation. Oxidation occurs as oxygen is metabolized in the body, which of course is a good thing, but oxidation can also damage cell membranes and DNA, accelerating the aging process. To see oxidation with your own eyes, cut an apple in half and observe it an hour later. The brown decay on the inside of the apple is caused by oxidation.

Antioxidants reverse the decay of oxidation by deactivating unstable free radicals. Natural antioxidants include vitamin C, vitamin E, and beta-carotene. By bringing the number of free radicals to a normal, more acceptable level, antioxidants control the aging process.

To test the antioxidant properties of cinnamon (_Cinnamomum verum_) and cardamom (_Amomum subulatum_), scientists in Pune, India, gave laboratory rats a high-fat diet that included cinnamon and cardamom. Then they studied the activity of the rats' antioxidant enzymes and glutathione (GSH). GSH is found in all human and animal cells and is a naturally occurring antioxidant. The scientists noticed increased activity among antioxidant enzymes in the rats. The rats' GSH content was "markedly restored." The scientists also reported that the cinnamon and cardamom appeared to counteract lipid peroxidation in the rats. Broadly defined, lipid peroxidation is the damage done by oxidation to polyunsaturated fatty acids in the body. Some have suggested that lipid peroxidation causes cardiovascular disease and kidney cancer.

By the way, antioxidants can be harmful if taken in excessive amounts. In a well-publicized study conducted in Finland, researchers found that the number of free radicals in smokers' lungs increased when they took the antioxidant beta-carotene. What's more, studies indicate that taking too much vitamin C actually encourages unnecessary free radicals to be released in the body. This is why the National Academy of Science recommends taking no more than one gram per day of vitamin C.

Antibacterial Effects of Cinnamon

Cinnamon is often an ingredient in toothpaste, chewing gum, and mouthwash for a very good reason. Besides tasting good, cinnamon can kill bacteria. Dental plaque, the substance that causes tooth decay, is made up of millions of bacteria. Bacteria buildup in the mouth is the chief cause of bad breath. Researchers have determined that cinnamaldehyde—one of the chemical components of cinnamon essential oil—is largely responsible for the antibacterial effects of cinnamon.

To measure the effect of cinnamon and cinnamaldehyde on different kinds of bacteria, scientists at National Taiwan University undertook experiments involving oil from the leaves of *Cinnamomum osmophloeum* and nine bacterial strains. The scientists concluded that the cinnamon essential oil and especially cinnamaldehyde had "excellent inhibitory effects." This table shows the results of the experiment. In the table, MICs (minimum inhibitory concentrations) are measured in micrograms per milliliter. The table shows the minimum amount of cinnamon oil or cinnamaldehyde that was needed to kill the bacterium or inhibit its growth. This experiment demonstrates that cinnamon is a fairly potent antimicrobial as well as a seasoning for food.

ANTIBACTERIAL EFFECTS OF CINNAMON			
BACTERIA	EFFECTS OF BACTERIA	CINNAMON OIL LEAF MICs (MICROG/ML)	CINNAMALDEHYDE MICs (MICROG/ML)
Enterococcus faecalis	Can cause urinary tract infections and wound infections.	250	250
Escherichia coli (E. coli)	Depending on the strain, can cause cramps and bloody diarrhea.	250	500
Klebsiella pneumoniae	Can cause pneumonia, burn wound infections, and hospital-acquired urinary tract infections.	500	1,000
Methicillin-resistant Staphylococcus aureus (MRSA)	Can cause boils, impetigo, and wound infections (and is resistant to some antibiotics).	250	250
Pseudomonas aeruginosa	Can cause respiratory tract, wound, eye, and ear infections. Cystic fibrosis sufferers, burn victims, and cancer patients are especially susceptible.	250	1,000
Salmonella	Can cause salmonella poisoning (cramps, diarrhea), severe headaches, nausea, vomiting, and low-grade fever.	500	500
Staphylococcus aureus	Can cause boils, impetigo, soft-tissue infections, and wound infections.	250	250
Staphylococcus epidermidis	Can cause skin irritations and is a common cause of many nosocomial (hospital-acquired) infections.	250	250
Vibrio parahaemolyticus	Can cause gastrointestinal illness.	250	250

Cinnamon versus Benzoic Acid

The next time you're reading the ingredients label on a food package, look for benzoic acid. Because of its antiseptic properties, benzoic acid is often an ingredient in packaged food. It keeps yeasts, bacteria, and microbes from growing and spoiling products. Benzoic acid is also blended into mouthwashes, shampoos, and cosmetics because it is so good at killing microbes.

Benzoic acid has been used as a preservative for centuries. It was originally isolated from benzoin gum, also known as gum benjamin, a resinous balsam that was used to make incense. The substance is found naturally in cloves, apples, plums, cranberries, and cinnamon.

In 1990, scientists at the Wuhan Institute of Traditional Chinese Medicine undertook a comparison of benzoic acid, beefsteak plant (*Perilla frutescens*), cinnamon (*Cinnamomum cassia*), and Nipagin A (methyl phydroxy-benzoate, a commercial mold inhibitor and anti-fungicide) as antimicrobials. The results of the experiment showed that the essential oil from cinnamon was "obviously superior" to Nipagin A and benzoic acid. This experiment demonstrates how powerful cinnamon is as an antimicrobial and the uses to which it can be put by the food industry.

Cinnamon and Respiratory Tract Mycoses

Respiratory tract mycosis is a fungal infection of the respiratory tract. The disease usually occurs in the lungs. It can cause mild flulike symptoms, fatigue, cough, fever, and chest pains. Respiratory tract mycosis is spread by airborne fungal spores. After a spore is inhaled, it changes into a larger, multicellular structure called a spherule. As the spherule grows, it may burst and release endospores in the lung, which in turn develop into more spherules, with the result being a full-blown fungal infection.

Most people do not need to concern themselves with respiratory tract mycosis. In a healthy immune system, the fungal spores are killed before they can cause infection or trigger an allergic reaction. But AIDS patients, older people, and others in whom the immune system is compromised are subject to infection from airborne fungal spores. Farmers, construction workers, and people who disturb the soil as part of their livelihood have a higher risk of being infected, but only if they live in areas such as the San Joaquin Valley of California, where the fungi that cause respiratory tract mycosis are common. (In the San Joaquin Valley, the fungus *Coccidioides immitis* causes a disease of the lungs known as Valley Fever.)

Cinnamaldehyde is known to be toxic to fungi. Using cinnamaldehyde, scientists in India conducted experiments on several of the fungi that cause respiratory tract mycosis. The scientists were interested in determining whether the bark oil from cinnamon, with its high cinnamaldehyde content, could be inhaled as a means of preventing fungal infections in the lungs. In the experiments, the following fungi were exposed to cinnamaldehyde in the test tube:

- *Aspergillus* (species *niger, fumigatus, nidulans,* and *flavus*). These fungi cause pulmonary aspergillosis and rhinosinusitis.

- *Candida* (species *albicans, tropicalis,* and *pseudotropicalis*). These fungi cause Candida oropharyngeal and esophageal candidiasis (as well as vaginal infections and thrush).

- *Histoplasma capsulatum.* This fungus causes histoplasmosis, also known as Darling's disease. It is found in the southern United States and South America. The fungus grows in soil that has been contaminated with bird or bat droppings.

The scientists reported that inhalable vapors from the bark oil of cinnamon appear to approach the ideal chemotherapy for respiratory tract mycosis. In other words, the cinnamaldehyde used in the experiment was entirely successful in inhibiting the growth of the fungi. It appears that inhaling essential oil made from the bark of cinnamon may be a way to prevent fungal infections in the lungs.

Cinnamon and Allergies

An allergy is a disease involving the immune system going into overdrive. Allergies are associated with antibodies of a class called IgE. When someone who is prone to allergies encounters an allergen for the first time, the person's B cells produce large numbers of antibodies of the type that are designed to counteract the allergen. The antibodies attach themselves to mast cells in the nose, tongue, skin, and gastrointestinal tract. The next time the person encounters the allergen, the body believes it is being attacked, and it may initiate an allergic reaction. The mast cells of the tissues team up with cells from the bloodstream—basophils and eosinophils—to release substances that create an acute inflammatory reaction. Outward signs of allergies include skin rashes, sneezing, watery eyes, runny nose, and even vomiting. Sometimes various organs are affected and begin to malfunction.

Researchers do not know exactly why one person gets an allergy and the next person doesn't. Allergies often run in families. Sometimes the environment makes a person more sensitive to allergens. For example, living with a cat can make a child sensitive to the cat's fur. Eating a diet too high in dairy products can cause the immune system to overreact.

In an experiment conducted in Japan, an aqueous extract of *Cinnamomum cassia* was tested in vitro on allergic reactions. The researchers found that the extract inhibited complement-dependent allergic reactions. In other words, cinnamon may be useful against angioedema, urticaria, and allergic reactions to drugs that cause body tissues to swell as a result of action by complement proteins.

Cinnamon, Candidiasis, and Oral Thrush

Infection with or disease caused by the yeast fungus *Candida albicans* is called candidiasis. As a yeast, *Candida albicans* is found on the skin and in the throat, mouth, digestive tract, and vaginal tract. If the yeast grows out of control, it can turn from a harmless yeast into an aggressive fungus and cause intestinal problems, vaginal infections, and an infection of the mouth and throat called thrush. To treat candidiasis and thrush, doctors prescribe antifungal agents called azoles. Azoles work by puncturing the membranes of fungal cells and killing them. Among AIDS patients, thrush and candidiasis have become serious problems in recent years. AIDS patients have weakened immune systems, which makes them more susceptible to candidiasis and thrush. What's more, some strains of *Candida albicans* are resistant to azole drugs.

In a trial conducted in Brooklyn in 1996, doctors at the Veterans Affairs Medical Center undertook an experiment to see if a commercially prepared cinnamon preparation could work against fluconazole-resistant thrush (fluconazole is a type of azole). In the trial, five patients infected with the HIV virus took the cinnamon preparation for one week. Three of five patients saw an improvement in their thrush. It appears that cinnamon's antifungal properties extend to *Candida albicans* as well as to other fungi.

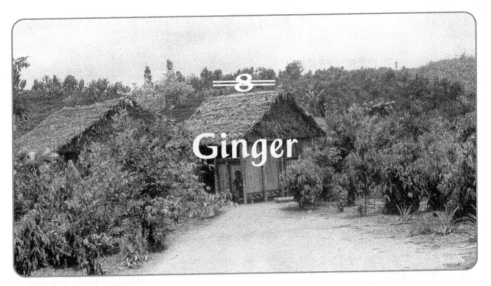

Ginger

inger (*Zingiber officinale*) is cultivated for its essential oil, for its oleoresin, and for use (fresh or dried and powdered) in baking and cooking. Malagasy ginger comes in two varieties: The blue-gray gingerroot, which is excellent for essential oil and oleoresin extraction, and the yellow gingerroot, which is for use in the kitchen.

Ginger essential oil is extracted by steam distillation from the fresh or dried root of the ginger plant. It is pale yellow to yellow-green in color. Oil made from dried ginger is darker, and all ginger oil tends to darken with age. The essential oil doesn't give off the pungent aroma most people are familiar with from cooking with ginger. Instead, it is subtler; it emits a fresh, clean smell and is warming, fortifying, antiseptic, spicy, and soft. Perfumers use it to give the feeling of warmth to perfume. Its lemony scent and peppery aura make it a popular ingredient in men's cologne and toiletry products. Tom's of Maine, a manufacturer of personal hygiene products, uses Malagasy fresh ginger oil in its "gingermint" toothpaste; the oil's appealing citrus note gives the toothpaste a unique zest.

Ginger oleoresin is a thick brown paste obtained by solvent extraction from the fibrous interior of the rhizome. The pungency of ginger is preserved in the oleoresin, which is why food manufacturers make use of it. It is often used to flavor soft drinks and medicine. Due to its poor solubility in alcohol, ginger oleoresin is not used in perfumes.

The name *ginger* comes from the Sanskrit *srngaveram*, which means "antler root," a reference to the rhizome's shape. En route to being called *ginger*, the plant was known to the Greeks as *ziggiberis*, to the Romans as *zinziberi*, and to early English speakers as *gingivere*. Ginger has the dis-

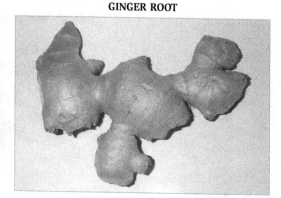
GINGER ROOT

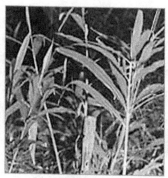
GINGER PLANT

tinction of being a verb as well as a noun. To "ginger up" means to make something a little livelier. The adverb "gingerly" means to act with alertness and care.

INTRODUCING THE GINGERROOT, OR RHIZOME

Technically, "gingerroot" is not the correct term for the ginger with which we are familiar. Ginger oil—and the ginger used in cooking and baking as well—comes from the plant's rhizome, not its roots. A rhizome, sometimes known as a rootstock, is a stem that grows underground. Shoots grow from its top and roots from its bottom. Rhizomes produce buds. On the ginger rhizome, the buds are the stubby, fingerlike protrusions (for this reason, the rhizome is sometimes called a "hand of ginger"). Buds from a rhizome grow if they are cut away from the rhizome and replanted in the soil. Irises, autumn ferns, horse radish, quickgrass, golden root, Kentucky bluegrass, and buffalo grass are other examples of plants with rhizomes.

The gingerroot is starting to make an appearance in grocery stores in the United States. It is a stumpy, gnarled, knobby, bulbous item that has the look of something that is good for you. Its skin is smooth, corky, and light brown. Most Americans know ginger as the powder in their spice racks, but you are hereby encouraged to include fresh ginger in your diet. Peel the rhizome's skin and either grate the ginger or slice it thinly. Small amounts of grated ginger add flavor to noodles, marinades, sauces, and curries. Ginger slices enliven soup stocks and herbal teas. Ginger slices steeped in hot water and flavored with honey may be the world's most popular folk remedy for the common cold. Do not store the rhizome in the refrigerator, where it may grow mold. Instead, store gingerroot at room temperature. Fresh ginger sometimes sprouts buds. These buds are considered a delicacy in parts of Asia.

Ginger prefers a hot, humid environment. In Madagascar, the plant is cultivated in the highlands and the central eastern regions, mostly in Beforona and its surrounding districts. It is also grown in India, China, Jamaica (the source of most powdered ginger), Nigeria, Sierra Leone, Fiji, and Australia. A small crop is grown in Hawaii and south Florida. (The "wild ginger" that grows in North America and sometimes goes by the name Canadian snakeroot or Indian ginger—its botanical name is *Asarum canadense*—is not related to real ginger.) About 100,000 tons of ginger is grown annually, and half of that crop is consumed in India. The United States imports 5,000 tons each year. Most of it is ground into powdered ginger for commercial baking.

THE CHEMISTRY OF GINGER

About 300 different chemical compounds are found in ginger. For the purpose of extracting ginger oil and oleoresin, the most important compounds are found in the tissue directly under the skin and in the fibrous interior of the rhizome. As we've mentioned, ginger essential oil is obtained by steam distillation, and ginger oleoresin by solvent extraction. Compounds in ginger oil (1 to 3 percent of the fresh rhizome) include zingiberene, bisabolene, and the citrals geranoil, limonene, and neral. Compounds in the oleoresin include gingeroles, zingerone, and shogaol (a word that means "ginger" in Japanese). They give ginger its pungent spiciness and are the most important medicinal components of ginger.

Ginger contains two enzymes, lipase and protease, that aid in digestion. Lipase breaks down fat and protease breaks down protein so it can pass through the wall of the small intestine and enter the bloodstream as nourishment. These important enzymes are also produced by the pancreas. Including ginger in your diet takes some of the burden away from your pancreas; it doesn't have to work as hard to create digestive enzymes because the enzymes are already present in the ginger. Asian chefs understood this principle intuitively and included ginger in their dishes to help with digestion as well as to improve flavor.

CULTIVATING AND HARVESTING GINGER AND GINGER OIL

Ginger is a hot-weather crop, but the plant can be temperamental. It favors a hot, moist climate and shade from the midday sun. It doesn't like tropical or dry heat and can't abide dry soil at all. For this reason, ginger is grown on small plots, often with a ground cover of mulch or leaves to help the soil retain its moisture.

More so than for other plants, soil quality has an enormous effect on ginger. Perhaps because its main growth (the rhizome) occurs underground, ginger needs an abundance of soil nutrients to thrive. The plant draws many nutrients from the soil, including minerals, nitrogen, and potash. It depletes the soil quickly and has to be rotated more often than most crops. Madagascar's nutrient-rich soil has proven excellent for growing ginger. At 1.3 to 3.5 percent, the essential oil yield is higher from ginger grown in Madagascar than from ginger grown elsewhere.

The ginger crop is planted in November or December and may be harvested six to seven months later, when the plants' leaves turn yellow and start to dry. The longer the rhizomes stay in the ground, the more pungent and flavorful they become. Ginger destined for the produce market, for candied ginger, and for ginger syrups is harvested on the early side and has a mild, moist, lemony flavor. Ginger that will be processed for powder and essential oil is harvested late in the nine-month term so that the rhizomes have more time to hoard flavor from the soil and dry out. However, leaving the rootstocks in the ground presents a risk for growers because it may subject the ginger to root rot and other fungal infestations.

The skin of the rhizome has to be peeled if the ginger is to be dried and used for powder or ginger oil. Most of the essential oil is found just below the skin, in the underlying tissue. Rough peeling of the skin also removes some of the underlying tissue and, thus, some of the essential oil. Properly done, peeling—also called scraping or uncoating—is a laborious, time-consuming activity. Some have called peeling the skin but not the underlying tissue a lost art, but, to be fair, some producers can't afford to pay for the labor of carefully peeling the skin. Low wages in Madagascar make it possible for peeling to be done carefully, so that the full flavor of ginger isn't taken away with the skin.

After the skin is peeled, the ginger is either dried or sent straight to the distillery for essential oil extraction. If the ginger is to be dried, the rhizomes are cleaned, shorn of their roots, and left in direct sunlight for seven to ten days. Drying accents the pungent flavor of ginger while reducing the lemony flavor. Most steam-distillation of ginger takes place in the importing countries, not the producer countries. On average, the yield of ginger oil is estimated at 15 to 17 kilograms per ton.

A GINGER HISTORY

Ginger has been used for cooking and as medicine for so long that no one knows its true origin. It is native to China, southern India, and the Malay Peninsula. It became a feature of Chinese cuisine and Chinese medicine very early. In the *Pen Tsao Ching,* or *Great Herbal,* a pharmacopoeia written about 3000 B.C.E., the sage-emperor Shen Nung recommends ginger as a treatment for colds, chills, and leprosy. (According to legend, Shen Nung tested hundreds of herbs on himself until a poisonous herb killed him.) The Confucian Analects, written in the fifth century B.C.E., note that Confucius "was never without ginger when he ate." Archeologists who unearthed the tomb of the Chinese Princess of Tai in 1972 found bamboo cases and pottery jars holding ginger and other spices (the princess died about 170 B.C.E.).

The ancient Assyrians, Babylonians, Egyptians, and Persians are known to have spiced their food with ginger, and Alexander the Great is supposed to have brought ginger to Europe after he conquered Persia. At any rate, by the first century C.E. the Romans were flavoring their wine with ginger (unadulterated wine was considered barbaric). The Greek physician Dioscorides (circa 40–90 C.E.) described ginger as an antidote to poisoning and an aid to digestion. *De Re Coquinaria,* Apicius's famous Roman cookbook of the fourth century C.E., offered six recipes that included ginger. The Roman doctors who accompanied the legionnaires carried ginger in their medicine kits. Galen (129–210), the father of Western medicine, wrote this about ginger: "It creates heat powerfully, but not immediately at first contact with pepper." The trade routes of antiquity carried dried ginger powder and other spices from east to west, from China to Goa to Calicut and onward to Nineveh, Alexandria, and Rome.

Unfortunately for Europeans of the era, ginger (along with a number of other tasty spices) was lost to European cuisine during the Dark Ages. Arabs monopolized the spice trade during this period. The missionaries of Islam, following the trade routes, spread their faith eastward and simultaneously captured the spice trade. Mohammed, it is worth noting, was himself a spice trader. He married a wealthy widow who had made her fortune trading in spices.

In the late Middle Ages, Marco Polo (1254–1324) sparked a spice revival in Europe when he wrote about ginger and other spices in his journals. Soon ginger was traveling the Silk Roads again and was being used in Europe to flavor cakes, sweetmeats, and patties. Ginger became tremendously valuable; one pound of ginger was worth one sheep. Henry VIII himself recommended ginger as a remedy against the plague. His recommendation is supposed to have inspired English bakers to invent gingerbread. Henry's daughter Queen Elizabeth I, to amuse her courtiers, had likenesses made of them in gingerbread, and so the gingerbread man was born. Ginger was all the rage in fifteenth-century Europe. The English and Irish put it in beer and created ginger beer. Queen Isabella of Spain included ginger on the shopping list of items Columbus was to bring back from the East (instead of ginger, he brought back parrots, chili seeds, tomato seeds, crude cigars, and syphilis).

To break the eastern monopoly on ginger, the Spanish set up ginger plantations in Jamaica in the early sixteenth century. The crop was an instant success. It inspired the Portuguese to grow ginger in Brazil and in their African colonies. Today, ginger dishes are a mainstay of Brazilian and West African cuisine. Ginger dishes are popular in Madagascar as well. *Romazava*, a beef and vegetable stew in a thin ginger-spiced gravy, is the national meat dish.

From about the time of the Civil War until the early twentieth century, a ginger-based patent medicine called Jake (named after the Jamaican origin of its ginger) was popular in the United States. Like most patent medicines, Jake's primary ingredient was alcohol. The medicine enjoyed a certain popularity with people whose religious beliefs or county government forbade them from drinking alcoholic beverages but not alcoholic medicines. With the coming of Prohibition in 1920, Americans from all walks of life discovered the wonderful medicinal qualities of Jake and its 70 to 80 percent alcohol content. Distillers who had formerly manufactured alcoholic beverages started manufacturing Jake instead. Tragically, one manufacturer adulterated his Jake with dangerous amounts of triorthocresylphosphate (TOCP), a chemical that can cause cell death in the spinal cord. Between 50,000 and 100,000 people were paralyzed or partially paralyzed in 1931 with "ginger Jake paralysis," better known as "Jake leg." The medicine quickly lost its popularity and its market. The Jake leg debacle hastened the end of Prohibition.

Jake is now forgotten in America except as the subject of a handful of blues songs.

Most Americans think of ginger ale when they hear the word *ginger.* This beverage is often thought to have been invented in Ireland, but the drink that tickles the nose was actually created in Toronto by a chemist named John McLaughlin, who made it in his soda water bottling plant in 1904. McLaughlin wanted to make a nonalcoholic equivalent to sparkling white wine. He named his new beverage "Canada Dry Ginger Ale." The drink proved so successful that he named his company after it. Canada Dry beverages, including ginger ale, are still sold in grocery stores.

GINGER OIL IN AROMATHERAPY

Aromatherapists recommend using ginger oil in combination with other essential oils because the oil by itself is too resolute. Ginger oil is thought to be especially bracing for the nerves. It is recommended in cases of anxiety and nervous tension. It sharpens the senses and can relieve fatigue and mental exhaustion. The oil's warming and uplifting fragrance is considered helpful in cases of frigidity and impotence. Some believe that ginger is an aphrodisiac.

Taken internally, a small drop of ginger oil helps digestion and relieves nausea, of course, but it also strengthens the appetite. For that reason, it is prescribed for anorexia. Ginger oil is said to improve blood circulation. It can be rubbed into the skin to alleviate varicose veins and cellulite.

Ginger has a fiery nature. When applied to skin, it should always be mixed with other oils, and it should never be applied to sensitive skin. In Chinese medicine, ginger is believed to encourage menstruation. Some aromatherapists believe that women who use ginger oil when they are pregnant run the risk of having a miscarriage. To be safe, women who are pregnant should not use ginger oil.

MEDICINAL USES FOR GINGER

Ginger can be found in the pharmacopoeia of many Asian countries. In traditional Chinese medicine, ginger is believed to act as a kind of internal sauna. It expels dampness and stimulates the yang Qi (pronounced CHEE), the warm body energy that is associated with vitality and vigor. In the Chinese tradition, ginger is considered an antidote to shellfish poisoning and was included for that reason in many seafood dishes.

The *Charaka Samhita,* the oldest text of Ayurvedic medicine (the traditional medicine of India), praises ginger as "the universal medicine" and recommends it especially for arthritis and other inflammatory joint diseases, as well as for problems with digestion. Ginger is classified as a pungent herb in the Ayurveda system. Pungent herbs—cayenne and garlic also fall in this classification—awaken *agni* in the body. *Agni* in Sanskrit means "fire." According to traditional Indian medicine, *agni* snatches the essence from food and converts it into energy for the body. By awakening *agni,* ginger improves digestion and body metabolism.

Ginger is one of the world's preeminent folk medicines. Daniele Ryman, author of *Aromatherapy: The Encyclopedia of Plants and Oils and How They Help You,* describes a Pacific island where traditional healers chew ginger and spit it on patients' wounds to heal them. In New Guinea, ginger is spat into canoes to prevent their cargo from being lost on the water and spat onto the road at village entrances to ward off evil. In Malaysia and Indonesia, new mothers eat ginger soup for thirty days after childbirth to help them sweat out impurities. Soda crackers and ginger ale is the folk remedy for an upset stomach in many American households.

Following are the results of some experiments undertaken to find out how ginger performs its magic and how it can be used to promote good health in modern times.

Ginger and Motion Sickness

You would never know it if you have been seasick, carsick, or airsick, but motion sickness begins in the brain and the inner ear, not the stomach. Certain nerve fibers of the vestibular system in the inner ear are responsible for keeping the body in balance. Motion sickness is caused by a difference of opinion between these nerve fibers and your vision. In a rocking boat, for example, your eyes tell your brain that the cabin walls are stable. Your eyes believe this because they are undulating at the same speed as the cabin walls. Meanwhile, the nerves of the inner ear that are responsible for balance scream that the whole world is tilting from side to side. These conflicting signals—all is stable, all is moving—confuse the brain and cause nausea, vomiting, and dizziness. The good news is that after a few days of this, the brain learns to understand and make sense of the conflicting signals. The bad news is that landing on terra firma again confounds the brain and causes another kind of confusion whereby the whole world seems heavier and more plodding than it used to.

Much anecdotal evidence suggests that ginger is useful against all forms of motion sickness. In some cultures, sailors chew raw ginger to keep from getting seasick. Ginger ale is often served on airplanes because it is known to prevent airsickness. Some people report that it works better than Dramamine. Ginger is also thought to support the digestive system and calm the stomach. It stimulates movement in the intestines and causes the salivary glands to produce more saliva. One of its compounds, galanolactone, blocks one of the chemicals that motivates vomiting. And between meals, ginger can prevent a reflux of the gastric juices. In other words, it can prevent stomach acids from rising into the esophagus and causing heartburn.

To see whether ginger's reputation as an aid to the stomach is not merely anecdotal, a number of studies have been done on ginger over the years.

- Scientists in Wüppertal, Germany, studied the effects of ginger on people who had just eaten. They discovered that ginger helps the stomach move downward (to be scientific, it helps gastroduodenal motility, the expansion and contraction of the stomach and beginning of the small intestine that plays a role in digestion). They also found that ginger helps prevent heartburn.

- Scientists at Kyoto Pharmaceutical University in Japan found a number of substances in ginger that demonstrate, at least in animals, some activity against stomach ulcers. Ulcers are also caused by a bacterium (*Helicobacter pylori*) that burrows into the lining of the stomach and causes inflammation. This bacterium, however, has its good points. It also prevents acid reflux, the splashing of stomach acids into the esophagus. It seems that people with stomach ailments can take their choice between having ulcers or heartburn, but not both or neither.

- In a double-blind placebo trial conducted on the North Sea, eighty Danish naval cadets were given one gram of powdered ginger or a placebo. Cadets who took powdered ginger suffered half as much seasickness—defined as cold sweats and the urge to vomit—as the placebo group did.

- In a ghastly study performed at Louisiana State University, twenty-eight unfortunate volunteers, electrodes attached to their abdomens, made "timed head movements" in rotating chairs until they reached the point of near vomiting. Then the volunteers were given powdered ginger, fresh ginger root, a placebo, or scopolamine, the drug derived from belladonna that sailors wear in a patch behind their ears to prevent seasickness. The subjects were asked to resume the timed head movements. We may judge from the results of the experiment that the outcome was rather messy and that ginger didn't do the trick this time. Subjects who took ginger vomited as often as the placebo subjects, performed on average the same number of jerky head movements, and demonstrated the same electrogastrogram activity. Subjects who took scopolamine fared better in all areas. (The twenty-eight students from Louisiana State University who volunteered for this experiment are to be commended for sacrificing so much of themselves for the advancement of medical science.)

Ginger and Nausea from Photopheresis

Photopheresis is a therapy used to treat cutaneous T-cell lymphoma (CTCL). This disease, a type of non-Hodgkin's lymphoma, is caused by malignant T cells. T cells are white blood cells that form the core of the immune system. In CTCL, the T cells grow uncontrollably on the skin. They can cause lesions and sometimes form tumors. Malignant cells can spread through the lymphatic system to other parts of the body. The tumor cells may also enter the bloodstream (a condition called the Sézary syndrome).

In photopheresis, a photosensitizing agent called 8-MOP (8-methoxypsoralen) is administered to the patient. Blood is then removed from the body through an intravenous (IV) line. The T cells in the blood are separated and exposed to ultraviolet light. This activates the 8-MOP in the T cells and alters the cells' DNA so they can't reproduce. Finally, the blood is returned to the body by reinfusion.

The procedure takes three to five hours. During that time, many patients experience extreme nausea. Knowing ginger's reputation for relieving nausea, doctors ran a clinical trial in which patients undergoing photopheresis were given ginger or a placebo. The patients who took ginger prior to taking 8-MOP reported a substantial reduction in nausea; the placebo patients reported no change. This trial shows yet again that ginger is helpful in preventing nausea. Other studies, however, have shown that taking ginger for postoperative nausea has no effect. Take your ginger before you go under the knife, not after.

Ginger and the Common Cold

What we call the common cold is caused by one of two hundred or so known viruses. About a third of colds are caused by a rhinovirus (from the Greek *rhin,* which means "nose"). There are 110 known rhinoviruses.

In the never-ending search for a cure to the common cold, scientists in England ran in vitro experiments to see whether the dried rhizome of Indonesian ginger can do the trick against a common strain of rhinovirus called rhinovirus IB. They isolated from the ginger several compounds thought to have antiviral activity and tested them against the virus in vitro. One compound, beta-sesquiphellandrene, proved especially effective against rhinovirus IB. Equally significant, only 0.44 microM of the compound was required. It appears that ginger is a potent inhibitor of at least one cold strain and that ginger therefore makes a good addition to the chicken soup you eat when you have a cold.

Ginger and Heart Attacks

To stop a cut from bleeding, platelets in the bloodstream stick to the part of the blood vessel that has been ruptured. The platelets clump together, or aggregate, at the site of the cut to form a kind of plug called a *thrombus.* Platelets are part of the body's healing mechanism. They prevent bleeding. However, platelets can be dangerous when they form blood clots along the artery walls of the heart. In this case, the clot can block the flow of blood to the heart. What's more, platelet clots can travel the arteries to other parts of the body. In the brain, they can cause strokes.

Animal fat in the diet tends to make platelets stick together more readily. This is one reason why you run the risk of having a heart attack if you eat too much fat. Recently, scientists in India and England undertook tests to see whether ginger can prevent platelets from clotting and thereby prevent heart attacks in people who eat a diet rich in animal fats.

- In a test at the Department of Medicine and Indigenous Drug Research Center in Udaipur, India, twenty male volunteers ate 100 grams of butter daily for a week. Butter is a very fatty substance. Half the volunteers were given 2.5 grams of dried ginger twice daily, in addition to the butter. An examination of this group's blood showed that platelet aggregation was inhibited.

• In a test conducted at the same research center under the same criteria, ginger caused *fibrinolytic,* or clot-dissolving, activity in volunteers who ate ginger as well as butter. This indicates that ginger can be useful in preventing blood clots.

• In a double-blind study at Harefield Hospital in Middlesex, England, eight male volunteers were fed butter as well as 2 grams of dried ginger or a placebo. After examining the volunteers' bleeding times and platelet counts, no difference was found between the placebo group and the group that ate dried ginger as well as butter. The English doctors concluded that fresh ginger, not the dried ginger they used in their experiment, is necessary to inhibit platelet aggregation. Moreover, two grams is not enough to effectively prevent blood clots.

These experiments seem to demonstrate that ginger can be useful in preventing heart attacks and blood clots. So if your cake contains butter, you can have it and eat it too, as long as fresh ginger is one of its ingredients.

Ginger and Mononucleosis

Ginger has been used as a folk remedy in Malaysia for many centuries. In 1999, Malaysian scientists conducted in vitro experiments to see whether the rhizome of Malaysian ginger can be useful against the Epstein-Barr virus (EBV). The virus is a member of the herpes family and is carried in the salivary glands. It is best known for causing infectious mononucleosis, known also as "mono." The disease causes swelling of the lymph glands, fever, fatigue, and a sore throat. The virus can also cause cancer of the nose, throat, and stomach. By age forty, nearly 90 percent of the population has contracted the virus, although most people do not acquire mononucleosis because their immune system keeps the virus in check. In their experiments, the Malaysian scientists discovered that ginger inhibits the growth of the EBV virus in the test tube and that compounds in ginger do not have any toxic activity. The authors of the study concluded that ginger might be useful against the types of cancer caused by EBV.

Ginger and Skin Cancer

Aging doesn't damage the skin; sunlight does. Sunlight is not just light and warmth. It is also composed of ultraviolet (UV) light. This kind of light can penetrate the skin and cause all kinds of damage to blood cells, nerves, and even the eyes. Long periods of exposure to ultraviolet light can damage the skin's DNA. When the DNA is damaged and cannot recover, it may degenerate, and the result can be skin cancer.

Recently, scientists at Case Western University ran tests to see whether an ether ethanol extract of ginger could inhibit damage from ultraviolet light and skin cancer as well. For the experiment, they applied the extract to the skin of laboratory mice that had skin tumors and mice with pre-cancerous skin conditions. They found that the ginger prevented the genesis and spread of the skin tumors. The experiment seems to indicate that ginger may be useful against certain kinds of cancer.

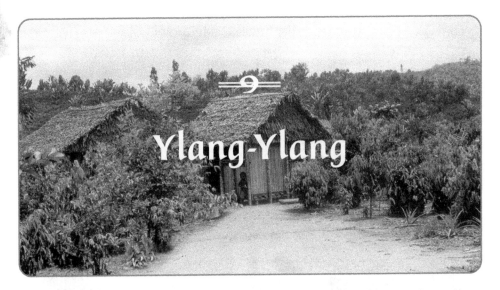

9

Ylang-Ylang

Ylang-ylang (pronounced EE'-lang EE'-lang) oil is made from the fragrant yellow flowers of the ylang-ylang tree (*Canaga odorata*). The name *ylang-ylang* comes from the Tagalog *álang-ilang*, which means "flower of flowers." In Malaysia, the ylang-ylang tree is known as the kananga, from which it derives its botanical name.

Madagascar and Mayotte, one of the nearby Comoro Islands, are now the leading producers of ylang-ylang essential oil. Soothing and sensuous, superior-grade ylang-ylang oil from Madagascar is flowery, sweet, soft, warm, and somewhat musky; perfumers and aromatherapists value it for its intense floral aroma and tenacity. Ylang-ylang has a slightly narcotic effect. The fragrance evokes deep-seated feelings of languor and calmness. Ylang-ylang essential oil is often blended into perfumes as a top or middle note. Thought to be the most romantic of essential oils, ylang-ylang has an aura of intimacy. The oil is exotic and alluring and has a reputation as an aphrodisiac.

Like so many other plants—among them vanilla, rose geranium, cinnamon, nutmeg, clove, and pepper—ylang-ylang was introduced to Madagascar by way of Réunion Island. Native to Indonesia, Malaysia, the Philippines, and other lowland countries of east Asia, the tall tropical tree is sometimes planted as an ornamental, because it provides abundant shade as well as its distinctive aroma. Although the ylang-ylang tree is not native to Madagascar, it flourishes in the volcanic soil and moist tropical climate of Nosy Bé, a 110-square-mile island off the northwest coast of Madagascar. Ylang-ylang has been cultivated in Nosy Bé, Nosy Komba, and the Ambanja region of Madagascar since 1905.

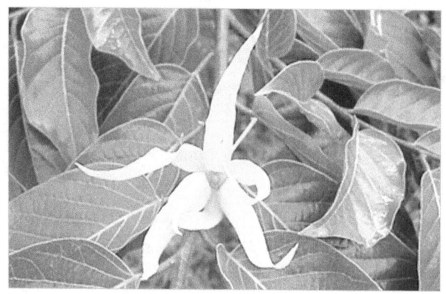

YLANG-YLANG

Nosy Bé, "the big island," is also known as Nosy Manitra, "the per-fumed island," because the odor of ylang-ylang flowers perfumes the air during the spring and summer. The island's coral reefs, excellent beaches, and reputation as a tropical paradise make Nosy Bé Madagascar's primary tourist destination.

YLANG-YLANG IN POMADES AND PERFUMES

Ylang-ylang has a long history of varied uses in the East and the West. In Indonesia, ylang-ylang flower petals are traditionally sprinkled on the bed of a newlywed couple on their wedding night. In the Philippines, ylang-ylang is used quite differently—in a salve to treat insect and snake bites. The inhabitants of the Molucca Islands crushed the flower petals and mixed them with coconut oil to form a hair pomade. Likewise, in Victorian England, gentlemen slicked back their hair with Rowland's Macassar oil, a pomade whose primary ingredient was ylang-ylang.

Macassar oil was named for Makasar, now Ujung Pandang, the former Dutch capital of Celebes, now Sulawesi. Macassar oil was supposed to promote hair growth as well as keep hair in place, and was applied duti-fully by both women and men. The well-groomed Victorian gentleman, his hair plastered down with Macassar oil, was redolent with the fragrance of ylang-ylang when he appeared in public. The oil was so popular in Victorian England that it gave rise to the antimacassar, a decorative covering folded over the top of upholstered chairs to keep the chairs from being stained by Macassar oil. Similarly, women in Victorian times took to wearing nightcaps in bed to keep their pillowcases and sheets from being stained.

Ylang-ylang essential oil today is used in cosmetics, soaps, face powders, and commercial fruit flavors, especially peach and apricot. Grade 3 ylang-ylang oil (we'll explain the grading system shortly) is also found in soaps and toiletry products.

The oil's best use may well be as an ingredient in popular perfumes. It is blended into Beautiful by Estée Lauder, Poison by Christian Dior, Champs-Elysées by Guerlain, Acqua di Gio by Armani, and Escape by Calvin Klein. Ylang-ylang is also a floral top note in the bestselling perfume of all time, Chanel No. 5.

CULTIVATING AND HARVESTING YLANG-YLANG OIL

Fragrant, star-shaped, yellow ylang-ylang flowers grow in clusters from the long, drooping branches of the ylang-ylang tree. In the wild, the tree can grow to 60 feet (20 meters), but cultivated trees are topped and their branches bent down to make harvesting the flowers easier. A tree does not produce flowers until its fifth year, after which it yields 45 pounds (20 kilograms) of flowers annually for a period of forty-five to fifty years.

The quality of ylang-ylang oil has a lot to do with how and when the flowers from which it is made are harvested. Ideally, flowers are harvested in the fall (soon after the rainy season ends in April, May, or June) and again in the spring (in October and November). Ylang-ylang flowers harvested during the rainy season are heavy with moisture and contain less essential oil. The flowers on some trees, however, can be harvested all year round, and to fill contracts some producers harvest when the essential oil is not at its highest level or its best.

The harvest begins when the flowers turn from green to a rich, golden yellow. Skilled hands are needed to harvest ylang-ylang flowers. Because the essential oil content is highest at night, field hands harvest the flowers in the cool morning hours, starting at daybreak. They must be careful to pick fully mature yellow flowers, not green flowers with low-quality essential oil. They must also handle the flowers carefully to keep them from being damaged in the containers, as damaged flowers can spread bacterial fermentation to other flowers. If the flowers can't be steam-distilled right away, they are spread carefully on the floor. Producers without enough floor space, however, have to leave the flowers in their containers and run the risk of the flowers fermenting and spoiling.

Ylang-ylang essential oil is made by steam distillation. Fifty pounds of ylang-ylang flowers are required to produce one pound of oil. The oil ranges in color from clear to light amber to yellow-brown; the higher the grade, the deeper the color. The scent of high-quality oil has a rich, flowery top note, whereas cheaper oils are cloying in high concentrations. Ylang-ylang oil must be stored carefully, because it quickly loses its fragrance when exposed to light.

Fractional Distillation

Ylang-ylang is one of the few essential oils that is produced by fractional distillation. In the course of the fifteen-hour steam distillation, oil is taken off the still in batches. The first batch, taken one hour into the distillation process, is called Extra grade or Extra fraction oil. Extra grade is the highest quality ylang-ylang oil and is coveted by the perfume industry. Subsequent grades are called First (taken after four hours), Second (at about seven hours), Third (about ten hours), and Complete (fifteen hours). Sometimes the Complete grade is a blend of the other grades rather than a complete distillation of the ylang-ylang flowers. First and Second grades are used for cosmetics; Third is used to scent soaps and skin-care products.

Extra and First grade exhibit the heaviest, most floral odor because they are rich in esters and linalool. The esters in these high-grade oils are responsible for ylang-ylang's soothing, antidepressant qualities. As you go down the line, the oils' fragrance becomes lighter and less floral. Because lower-grade ylang-ylang oils are low in esters and high in sesquiterpenes, they are the better choice for skin-care products.

Canaga oil, similar to but less perfumed than ylang-ylang oil, is made from the tree *Canaga adoratum*. Ylang-ylang comes from *Canaga odorata*. Don't confuse these essential oils. Canaga oil is sometimes blended into cheaper perfumes. It doesn't have the potency or tenacity of ylang-ylang.

YLANG-YLANG IN AROMATHERAPY

Due to its reputation as an aphrodisiac and sexual stimulant, ylang-ylang is often recommended by aromatherapists in cases of impotence and frigidity. To make the most of ylang-ylang's properties as an aphrodisiac, the aromatherapist Jeanne Rose suggests scenting cotton balls with the oil and placing them in the dresser drawer where the lingerie is kept.

Ylang-ylang oil is thought to be an antidepressant. Aromatherapists prescribe it to lower blood pressure and relieve the effects of nervousness and stress. A few drops in a warm bath can be very relaxing. It is also said to relieve insomnia, PMS, and the uncomfortable side effects of menopause.

Rubbing ylang-ylang oil into your hair is a good remedy for dry scalp. Ylang-ylang, however, should always be diluted with a carrier oil. It is usually blended with lemongrass, sandalwood, patchouli, or orange essential oils. Because ylang-ylang is such a strong fragrance, it can cause nausea and headaches if it is not used in moderation.

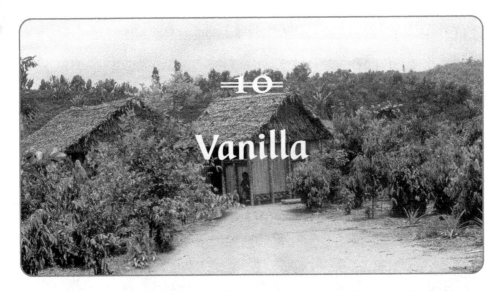

10

Vanilla

Most people know vanilla as an ice cream flavor and a baking ingredient, but vanilla is more than a flavor. It is also a fragrance. Perfumers use vanilla as a base or middle note because its rich, sweet aroma is long-lasting and it complements other aromas. Most perfumes contain at least a small amount of vanilla, and it is the base note in one-third of all perfumes. Vanilla is also found in most chocolate. It is an ingredient in house paint, rubber tires, and household cleaning products, where it is used to disguise unpleasant chemical odors. Vanilla flavoring is added to medicines to make them more palatable. It can be found in soaps, body lotions, shampoos and conditioners, deodorants, candles, body lotions, massage oil, and incense.

Vanilla has a seductive charm and a certain erotic component. The fragrance is intimate and elusive. Compared to most essential oils, vanilla is understated. It works its magic slowly but surely. Because it sees so much use in baking, the scent of vanilla conjures happy associations in many people. For many, vanilla represents the comforts and warmth of home. In an ice cream parlor that offers exotic tropical flavors and all manner of sugary confections, many choose the soothing taste of vanilla. Vanilla does not deserve the "plain" tag that is sometimes attached to it in the United States. There is nothing "plain" about "plain vanilla." Vanilla is subtle and bewitching, not plain.

Vanilla is derived from fruit—it resembles a long green bean—of the tropical orchid. Of the twenty thousand species in the orchid family, only two hundred or so produce a bean. And of the two hundred fruit-bearing species, only two, Bourbon (*Vanilla planifolia* Andrews, sometimes known

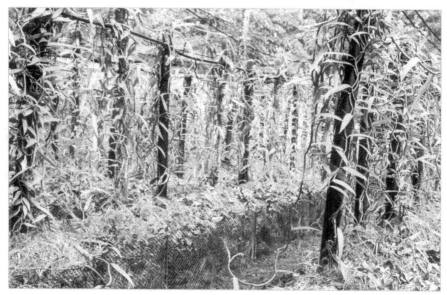

VANILLA

as *Vanilla fragrans* Ames) and Tahitian (*Vanilla tahitensis* Moore), are used for the commercial production of vanilla. The tropical orchid grows on a thick vine. Except for its yellow or orange flower, it does not resemble the garden-variety orchid most people know.

Connoisseurs of vanilla agree that the most delicious beans come from Madagascar and the Comoro Islands. Their tropical climate, tempered by cooling marine breezes from the Indian Ocean, and the combination of a half-year hot and dry season followed by a half-year rainy season seem to bring out the best in vanilla beans. They are richer and moister than vanilla beans grown elsewhere, with a sweet, creamy, aromatic flavor.

THE HISTORY OF VANILLA

Vanilla has a long and storied history. The tropical orchid is one of those plants, like the potato and tobacco, that have altered the course of history. From its discovery in Mexico, vanilla traveled to all four corners of the world, including Madagascar. Madagascar is now the world's leading producer of natural vanilla.

Vanilla in the New World

The history of vanilla begins in the Kingdom of Totonocopan, located in the Mazantla Valley on the Gulf Coast of Mexico near present-day Vera Cruz. At some time in prehistory, the Totonaca people who inhabited the kingdom and still live in the Vera Cruz region discovered how to cultivate vanilla beans from the tropical orchid. They revered vanilla as the "nectar of the gods." According to Totonaca mythology, the tropical orchid was born when Princess Xanat, forbidden by her father from marrying a mortal, fled to the forest with her lover. The lovers were captured and beheaded. Where their blood touched the ground, the vine of the tropical orchid grew. Traditional healers among the Totonaca used vanilla to cure stomach ailments, coughs, and respiratory problems. To this day, the Totonaca perfume their homes with vanilla, wear the beans in their hats for fragrance, and dangle vanilla beans from the rear-view mirrors of their cars as a talisman.

In the fifteenth century, Aztecs from the central highlands of Mexico conquered the Totonaca, and the conquerors soon developed a taste for the vanilla bean. They named the bean *tlilxochitl,* or "black flower," after the mature bean, which shrivels and turns black shortly after it is picked. Whereas most tribes paid tribute to the Aztecs in the form of maize or gold, the Totonaca sent vanilla beans to the Aztec kings. Vanilla became a favorite of the Aztec nobility. In the royal court, it was considered an aphrodisiac. The Aztecs mixed vanilla into *chocotatl* (alternate spellings are *tlilxochitl* and *xoco-latl*), known otherwise as chocolate, a drink made from cocoa beans that the Aztecs learned to prepare from the Mayas. King Montezuma of the Aztecs is supposed to have drunk *chocotatl* for inspiration before visiting his wives' bedchambers. Techniques devised by the Aztecs for fermenting and curing vanilla beans are still used today.

The Europeans who arrived on the Gulf Coast of Mexico in the early sixteenth century soon discovered the vanilla bean and its seductive charm. They recognized vanilla as a candidate for an essential oil. They knew immediately that it could be a valuable ingredient in perfumes. Vanilla beans were dispatched to Spain for study.

Meanwhile, Hernando Cortés, the Spanish conqueror of the Aztecs, became the first European to taste vanilla when he drank *chocotatl* in Montezuma's banquet hall. In his epic *The Discovery and Conquest of Mexico,* Bernal Díaz, a soldier who accompanied Cortés, relates how Montezuma served *chocotatl* in golden goblets with turtle shell spoons. The chocolate that Montezuma served, by the way, was not sweet. It was made from cocoa beans, ground corn, chili, allspice, and vanilla. The Spanish added sugar and cinnamon to chocolate when they started manufacturing it in the sixteenth century.

The Spanish called the bean *vainilla*, or "little pod," because the slender vanilla bean reminded them of the green bean and its pod. One wonders, however, if the Spanish had the orchid's appearance or vanilla's reputation as an aphrodisiac in mind when they named vanilla. *Vaina* in Spanish means "vagina" (*vaina*, as well as the English *vagina*, comes from the Latin word for "sheath"). The word *vanilla* entered the English language in 1754, when botanist Philip Miller wrote about the genus in his *Gardener's Dictionary*. Miller anglicized the Spanish *vainilla* by dropping the first *i* from its name.

Vanilla Goes to Europe

Vanilla quickly became a favorite in Europe, especially in France. By the end of the sixteenth century, factories for producing vanilla-flavored chocolate had been established throughout Spain. Soon vanilla came into its own as a flavoring and fragrance. It was used in perfumes, baking, snuff, liqueurs, and pipe tobacco.

The tropical orchid became an object of curiosity among European botanists. Hugh Morgan, the apothecary to Queen Elizabeth I, is thought to be the first European to suggest using vanilla as a flavor by itself. In 1602, Morgan sent cured vanilla beans to the Flemish botanist Charles de l'Écluse (also known as Carolus Clusius), who described them in his *Exoticorum Libri Decem* (*Book of Many Exotic Plants*), an authoritative work that introduced Europeans to exotic plants from the New World, including tobacco, the avocado, and the potato. Vanilla also made an appearance in the other well-known book about New World plants from the period, *Rerum Medicarum Novae Hispaniae Thesaurus*, published in Rome in 1651. This book was written by Francisco Hernandez, a Spanish physician who conducted research on the flora and fauna of Mexico for Philip II.

None other than Thomas Jefferson brought vanilla to the shores of the United States. After his return to America in 1789, the former ambassador to France and future president of the United States, an admirer of French cuisine as well as French philosophy, craved the taste of vanilla. He wrote to the American chargé d'affaires in Paris and received fifty vanilla beans. Jefferson is supposed to have served vanilla ice cream in the

White House. In the Jefferson Papers collection in the Library of Congress is a recipe for vanilla ice cream written in Jefferson's own hand (on the other side of the card is a recipe for Savoy cookies).

Vanilla Comes to Madagascar

Vanilla was extremely expensive in nineteenth-century Europe. It was grown only in Mexico. And until the middle of the nineteenth century, Mexico had vanilla production all to itself. The Vera Cruz region, site of the world's only vanilla cultivation, prospered. All vanilla had to come from Mexico.

French entrepreneurs and horticulturalists knew that they could make a fortune by cultivating vanilla outside Mexico. If they broke the Mexican monopoly, they could exploit vanilla's high price and turn a tidy profit. The appetite for vanilla among the French was, and still is, enormous. French horticulturalists turned their attention to two tropical islands in the southwest corner of the Indian Ocean where they believed vanilla could be cultivated: Réunion and Mauritius, then known as the Bourbon Islands. The climate and soil composition of these islands was similar to that of Vera Cruz. If you could grow the tropical orchid in Mexico, the French reasoned, you could also grow it in the Bourbon Islands.

Tropical orchids were shipped to Réunion Island in 1819. Much to the delight of horticulturalists, the plants prospered. However, the orchids failed to produce a single ripe pod. The vines flowered, but they did not produce any vanilla beans.

Charles Morren, a professor of botany at the University of Liège in Belgium, solved the mystery of why the vanilla orchid could not bloom on the Bourbon Islands. The problem, it turned out, had to do with the absence of natural pollinators. In its native Mexico, the Melipona bee pollinates the tropical orchid and allows it to bear fruit. (Hummingbirds have been observed visiting the orchids, and some have suggested that hummingbirds may also be a pollinating agent.) Outside of Mexico, however, insects have no interest in the tropical orchid. On the Bourbon Islands, the flowers fell from the vine almost as soon as they bloomed because no insect would pollinate them. Although the vines thrived, they were sterile.

To solve the pollination problem, horticulturalists attempted to introduce the Mexican Melipona bee to Réunion Island, but their experiment failed. The vanilla orchid would have to be pollinated by hand if it was to be pollinated at all. In 1836, Charles Morren developed a method of hand-pollinating the tropical orchid.

Morren's method, however, was slow and required too much effort to make cultivating vanilla a moneymaking proposition. It remained for Edmond Albius, a former slave from Réunion Island, to invent a speedy method whereby the orchids could be pollinated quickly and profitably. The twelve-year-old boy discovered how to pollinate the vanilla orchid with a thin stick or blade of grass and a simple thumb gesture. With the stick or grass blade, field hands lift the rostellum, the flap that separates the male anther from the female stigma, and then, with their thumbs, they smear the sticky pollen from the anther over the stigma. Albius's manual pollination method is still used today. Nearly all vanilla is pollinated by hand. The procedure accounts for about 40 percent of the labor costs of producing vanilla. Hand-pollination, incidentally, represents an improvement over natural pollination because healthy vines can be made to bear more.

News of the successful pollination of a vanilla orchid spread across Réunion Island. It traveled as well to the other French possessions in the region. On Réunion Island, a failure of the sugar crop encouraged growers to try their hand at vanilla. In 1843, tropical orchids were sent from Réunion Island to the Comoro Islands and Madagascar along with instructions for pollinating them. Within a generation, these French colonies became the center of world vanilla production, the vanilla from *Vanilla planifolia* came to be called "Bourbon vanilla," and Bourbon vanilla became the favorite of vanilla connoisseurs. The first vanilla beans to be exported from the Bourbon Islands, fifty in all, were sent from Réunion Island to France in 1848. Fifty years later, in 1898, Madagascar, Réunion, and the Comoro Islands produced 200 metric tons of vanilla beans, about 80 percent of world production.

Most of this vanilla was produced on vast plantations owned by French or Créole colonists in northeast Madagascar near Antalaha. The plantations in this hot, rain-soaked region were worked by indentured Malagasies supplied on contract by the French colonial administration. When slavery was outlawed in 1896 (outlawing slavery was one of the first acts of the new colonial government), the French found themselves with a shortage of laborers for vanilla production. To solve the problem, they resorted to conscription, a technique used by the old kings and queens of

Madagascar. Starting with World War I and ending with the Great Depression, however, the plantation system fell into decline. Today, most vanilla from Madagascar is produced between Antalaha and Taomasina (Tamatave) on family holdings of the Betsimisaraka tribe (the name means "The Inseparable Many" in Malagasy).

Worldwide, the annual production of cured vanilla beans amounts to about 1,600 to 1,800 metric tons. Production varies due to weather conditions. Madagascar supplies about 35 percent of vanilla beans (down from 70 percent in the 1970s and 1980s). The majority of vanilla is consumed in the United States and Europe, where it is used mostly to flavor ice cream, yogurt, and other dairy products.

Vanilla is also grown in Indonesia, Tahiti, Costa Rica, Guatemala, Uganda, China, the Philippines, Fiji, Tonga, and Papua New Guinea. Mexico, vanilla's native land, produces very little of the world's vanilla. Vanilla cultivation in Mexico declined during the revolution of 1910 and has never recovered. What's more, oil production in the Vera Cruz region has raised wages and made the cultivation of vanilla too expensive. Sadly, the Totonaca, the original cultivators of vanilla, were expelled from their native lands in 1896. The Mexican government claimed that the Indians had no title to the land and sold it to others. Vanilla cultivation among the Totonaca has shrunk to a cottage industry.

IS VANILLA AN APHRODISIAC?

Unfortunately, science has yet to discover a universal aphrodisiac. What constitutes an aphrodisiac for one person leaves the next person completely indifferent. Nevertheless, the search for the universal aphrodisiac continues. At various times in different cultures, oysters, ginger, the shiitake mushroom, quince, rosemary, bananas, nutmeg, tiger penises, kumquats, marijuana, green M&Ms, licorice, and figs were thought to be aphrodisiacs. In eighteenth- and nineteenth-century Europe and America, more than a few physicians believed that vanilla was it. They believed that vanilla encouraged feelings of passionate amorousness and desire.

Chocolate, with vanilla as one of its ingredients, enjoyed a huge vogue in eighteenth- and nineteenth-century Europe. Chocolate's flavor, of course, accounted for its popularity, but chocolate's aphrodisiacal element also played a part. Chocolate manufacturers in Europe encouraged the idea that vanilla is an aphrodisiac. It was good for business. In the medical reasoning of the day, substances were categorized according to their coldness or heat, and vanilla was deemed very hot. Grooms were instructed to drink beverages flavored with vanilla on their wedding nights. In the court of Louis XV, vanilla was added to the chocolate to make the evenings livelier. The Comtesse du Barry, the mistress of Louis XV, is supposed to have remarked that vanilla is what kept Louis interested.

Physicians who believed in vanilla's reputation as an aphrodisiac sometimes prescribed vanilla for impotence or, as we call it today, erectile dysfunction. In his 1762 essay "On Experiences," German physician Bezaar Zimmermann wrote, "No fewer than 342 impotent men, by drinking vanilla decoctions, had changed into astonishing lovers of at least as many women." Dr. Zimmermann did not say how he conducted his study on the 342 men, how much vanilla they drank, or how many women they seduced altogether.

In *The American Dispensatory* (1859), an authoritative book that described some six hundred herbs and substances, president of the Eclectic Medical Association Dr. John King had this to say about vanilla:

Action, Medical Uses, and Dosage.—Aromatic stimulant. Vanilla is said to exhilarate the brain, prevent sleep, increase muscular energy, and stimulate the sexual propensities. Useful, in infusion, in hysteria, rheumatism, and low forms of fever. It is also considered an aphrodisiac, powerfully exciting the generative system. Much used in perfumery, and to flavor tinctures, syrups, ointments, confectionery, etc.

When vanilla extract came on the market at the end of the nineteenth century, poor Frenchwomen who could not afford expensive perfumes used vanilla instead, dabbing it on their wrists and behind their ears. These women knew that vanilla has a charm that men find appealing.

Vanilla's reputation as an aphrodisiac continues today. In parts of Latin America, for example, vanilla beans are dissolved in tequila, rum, or another clear alcohol to make an aphrodisiac concoction. Men who take ten to fifteen sips of the concoction each night are supposed to maintain their sexual vigor. Whether the vanilla-alcohol concoction really promotes sexual vigor is hard to say. The alcohol may delude the men into thinking they are virile. Alcohol does that sometimes.

CULTIVATING AND CURING VANILLA

Cultivating and curing vanilla is labor intensive. Only saffron and cardamom, it is said, require more labor to grow and produce than vanilla. The vines are grown from cuttings and do not bud until the third or fourth year. Unless the tropical orchids are pollinated on the day they bloom—and they must be pollinated by hand—they will die. Flowers bloom over a period of two months, so field hands must always be ready to hand-pollinate them. A flower that isn't pollinated on the day it blooms falls from the vine and does not produce vanilla beans. The beans are podlike and green. They resemble large green beans. Mature beans are a half-inch wide and four- to six-inches long.

In their natural state, tropical orchid vines creep to the top of the rainforest canopy. Workers have to train the unruly vines to grow on trellises. They have to trim unwanted buds, blossoms, and beans. The beans ripen for seven to nine months and are harvested when their tips turn golden yellow. The longer beans stay on the vine, the more concentrated their flavor will be, but a bean that is left on the vine too long may split during the curing process and have to be sold for vanilla extract. The curing process begins after the beans are harvested. As much as anything, curing determines how flavorful the beans are. The process lasts three to six months and is a high art that requires patience and care.

For a time, Madagascar's vanilla growers had to contend with vanilla rustlers, thieves who would enter the fields in the dead of night. Vanilla growers woke up in the morning to find that portions of their valuable crop had been stolen. To protect their crops, the growers came up with an ingenious solution—they branded the vanilla beans. Before the vanilla beans were ripe enough to pick, the growers carved distinctive markings on each bean with a pin. This practice put an end to vanilla rustling. The stolen beans were too easy to identify.

On the vine, the beans give off the distinctive aroma of vanilla. Interestingly, however, vanilla beans have no fragrance or flavor at harvest time. Only after the curing process do the beans reacquire the familiar vanilla smell.

In Madagascar, vanilla beans undergo the "Bourbon process," a superior curing technique named for the Bourbon Islands where the process was developed. Curing begins a week after the harvest and lasts three to six months. Slow, patient curing is what distinguishes the Bourbon process from other curing processes in which overdrying and rapid drying rob the beans of their moisture.

To halt photosynthesis and make the beans wilt, the newly harvested beans are submerged in hot water for several minutes. Next comes the sweating phase. By day, the beans are spread on blankets in the hot sun to bake; by night they are sealed in boxes. As the beans dry, they wrinkle, turn dark brown, and acquire the pungent vanilla aroma. Beans shrink by about 25 percent during the sweating phase. When the head curer decides that the beans are properly sweated, the conditioning phase begins. The beans are stored in holding rooms for several months. During this period, minute white spicules appear on the beans. This is the pure vanillin crystallizing as it oozes out of the pod.

Finally, the beans are ready to ship. High-grade beans are separated out. The beans are sorted by grade, size, and moisture content, then tied in bundles and packed in metal boxes. The ideal moisture content is 18 to 25 percent. Beans with too much or too little moisture lack the vanilla flavor. The conditioning phase continues for several months more as the vanilla beans travel to their final destinations.

Synthetic Versus Authentic Vanilla Extract

According to some estimates, 95 percent of the vanilla used in fragrances and flavoring is synthetic. German scientists began producing synthetic vanilla extract in the 1880s. The high cost of producing natural vanilla and the need for vanilla on the part of food manufacturers and industry created a market for the synthetic stuff.

Of the two hundred or more organic components found in natural vanilla, synthetic vanilla contains only one—vanillin. Vanillin is the primary component of vanilla. It is most responsible for vanilla's unique fragrance. Some synthetic vanilla extracts also contain propylene glycol, an ingredient in automotive antifreeze!

You can tell whether vanilla extract is synthetic or pure by looking at it. Authentic vanilla is the color of amber. Synthetic vanilla usually contains caramel coloring or ethyl, which causes it to have a dark tint.

Vanilla flavor can be manufactured from the tonka bean, which contains coumarin, a substance that smells like vanilla when it has been fermented. Coumarin is sometimes used in place of vanilla in perfumes, soaps, and foods. Unfortunately, coumarin is an anticoagulant, or anticlotting agent, that can cause serious bleeding. The substance is also a photosensitizer (it can cause rashes to develop if you are exposed to the sun after ingesting it). What's more, in high doses coumarin can cause liver and kidney damage.

Vanilla flavoring is also manufactured from clove oil and from lignin, a byproduct of paper manufacturing.

No matter what the labels say, most vanilla extract produced in Mexico, Central America, and South America is synthetic. Furthermore, much of it contains coumarin. Because Mexican labeling laws do not require ingredients to be listed on labels, determining how much coumarin is in vanilla extract is impossible. Writes Patricia Rain, the author of _Vanilla Cookbook_, "The fact is that label laws are non-existent or aren't enforced. These are poor countries taking advantage of Mexico's early reputation as the producer of the best vanilla in the world. Unless the bottle costs over $20 a quart and has 35 percent alcohol, it is not pure vanilla extract."

Tropical storms in the year 2000 and 2001 badly damaged Madagascar's vanilla crop and raised the price of vanilla dramatically. Seeking to take advantage of high prices and the vanilla shortage, producers in China and other Asian countries have been flooding the market with synthetic vanilla. Although the labels on these products claim that they are "natural," a word to the wise is sufficient. These products are made with synthetic vanillin produced in the laboratory.

Bourbon and Tahitian Vanilla

Previous to its cultivation in Madagascar, vanilla was grown in two other French colonies in the Indian Ocean: Réunion and Mauritius. These islands were formerly named the Bourbon Islands after the Bourbon kings of France. Bourbon vanilla, the type of vanilla grown in Madagascar, gets its name from the Bourbon Islands. However, Bourbon vanilla and the type of vanilla that was cultivated in ancient Mexico are one and the same. They come from the same plant stock. Most vanilla, with the exception of vanilla cultivated in Tahiti and the West Indies, is Bourbon vanilla.

Tahitian vanilla also comes from plant stock that originated in Mexico, but in the past sixty years, the Tahitian orchids have mutated and evolved into a different species. The new species is called Tahitian vanilla (_Vanilla tahitensis_ Moore). Tahitian vanilla is decidedly different from the Bourbon variety. It is damper and not as sweet. As with all things, which kind of vanilla is preferable is a matter of taste. Tahitian vanilla has become expensive of late because less of it is being grown in Tahiti, and Tahiti is the only place where it is cultivated.

The third type of commercial vanilla comes from *Vanilla pompona* Shiede, also known as Guadeloupe vanilla or Antilles vanilla, a tropical orchid native to the West Indies. Beans from this orchid mature faster than *Vanilla planifolia* beans, but they are dry and of poor quality. They are used exclusively for making vanilla extract.

By the way, the term "French vanilla" doesn't describe a type of vanilla. French vanilla is a custard base for ice cream. And it is also a favorite of copywriters, who find the term irresistible and apply it to all manner of things from clothing colors to aromatic candles to lipstick.

MEDICINAL USES FOR VANILLA

In nineteenth-century Europe, vanilla was used as a febrifuge, or a medicine for reducing fevers. Among the Totonaca people, the original purveyors of vanilla, the substance was used to treat congestion. Vanilla is an antacid, and until the turn of the previous century, pharmacists prescribed it for nausea and queasiness. Even Coca-Cola, because it contains a significant amount of vanilla, was prescribed for upset stomachs once upon a time. And because vanilla conjures happy childhood memories in some people, it has been used as an antidepressant.

Incidentally, vanilla makes a good insect repellent, according to Patricia Rain, author of *Vanilla Cookbook*. She suggests crushing one or two vanilla beans into furniture polish. Insects can't tolerate the smell of vanilla and, moreover, using vanilla in furniture polish leaves the house smelling very nice.

The following pages describe some medical trials that were conducted to test these and other medicinal uses associated with vanilla.

Vanilla and Anxiety

In 1991, psychologist Dr. Sharon Manne of New York's Memorial Sloan-Kettering Cancer Center ran an experiment to see whether vanilla's calming fragrance could help patients undergoing MRI (magnetic resonance imaging) tests. For many patients these tests are an unbearable ordeal. Patients must lie on a narrow table inside a tunnel-like tube. Tests last from sixty to ninety minutes. Most patients experience some degree of anxiety and some experience claustrophobia as well. An MRI test costs $1,500, so being able to complete an MRI is important.

For the experiment, doctors scented the air in the MRI room with heliotropin, a compound with a distinct vanilla odor. Dr. Manne reported a 63 percent decrease in anxiety among patients who breathed the vanilla aroma during their MRI tests. She speculated that vanilla's familiar, agreeable odor had a relaxing effect on her patients. Since the Sloan-Kettering experiment, other hospitals have adopted vanilla aromatherapy for MRI testing.

Vanilla and Weight Loss

Obviously, maintaining proper body weight is important for your health. According to the United States Centers for Disease Control, obesity—defined as being 30 percent or more above ideal body weight—increased from 12 percent of the population in 1991 to 17.9 percent in 1998.

In the year 2000, Catherine Collins, a dietician at St. George's Hospital in London, England, conducted a novel experiment to see whether vanilla could help people lose weight. Collins was concerned about the dangerous side effects of weight-loss drugs. She wanted to see whether vanilla, a natural ingredient, could be used in place of those drugs.

"We know that taste and aroma do have a feedback on brain biochemistry fairly immediately to tell you to stop eating," Collins said. "In psychology literature there has been a lot of work on this, but it has never been applied to obese patients before."

In the experiment, Collins selected two hundred overweight volunteers, divided them into three groups, and had them wear a vanilla patch, a lemon patch, or a patch with no fragrance for four weeks. The vanilla-patch group lost 4.5 pounds on average, whereas weight loss in the other two groups was negligible.

Interestingly, volunteers who wore the vanilla patch ate less chocolate and took fewer sugary drinks, although their intake of fatty foods, starches, and alcohol remained the same. Collins believes that the vanilla fragrance produced higher levels of serotonin in the volunteers' brains. Serotonin, a chemical neurotransmitter, is believed to suppress appetite and hunger.

"There is some research that shows very sweet smells release serotonin in the brain," she said. "Serotonin is a mood chemical that makes you feel good, which is why chocolate also has that effect. Its chemical content produces serotonin."

Vanilla patches under the trade name Crave Control can be purchased from the Aromacology Patch Company of West Yorkshire, England.

Vanilla and Male Erectile Dysfunction

The belief that some fragrances excite sexual desire is as old as the hills. Recently, Dr. Alan Hirsch, a neurologist and psychiatrist who directs the Smell and Taste Treatment and Research Foundation in Chicago, put this age-old belief to the test. For the experiment, Dr. Hirsch investigated various aromas to see how they affect the flow of blood to the penis. The purpose of the test was threefold:

- To find out which scents are arousing.

- To see whether aromas could be used to treat vasculogenic impotence, the inability to achieve an erection due to the obstruction of blood flow to the arteries of the penis. Some ten million American men are believed to suffer from impotence. For half of them, the problem is physiological, not psychological.

- To find out whether some scents discourage arousal. Dr. Hirsch wanted to see whether these scents could be used to treat sex offenders.

In the double-blind study, thirty-one volunteers tried on masks with different scents as well as masks with no scent at all. Scents included vanilla, strawberry, lavender, peppermint, cinnamon, doughnut (the doctor didn't report which flavor), roasting meat, and buttered popcorn. No odor decreased the flow of blood to the penis. Lavender was deemed most arousing. Men who reported having frequent sexual activity and men whose sexual partners wear perfume were most aroused by lavender. Vanilla, however, proved most arousing to older men. The moral: To snare an older, mature gentleman, someone with experience to his years and many assets in his financial portfolio, try wearing the scent of vanilla.

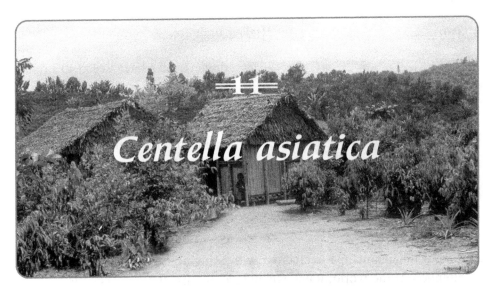

11

Centella asiatica

nlike the other plants we examine in this book, *Centella asiatica* does not produce an essential oil, but we include it here because extracts from the plant have proven very effective in pharmaceutical drugs and cosmetics. What's more, *Centella asiatica* has become an important plant of economic value to Madagascar. Pharmaceutical companies prize *Centella asiatica v. typica* from Madagascar because of its high concentration of triterpenoid compounds. Triterpenoids, also called triterpenes, are aromatic compounds that have interesting medicinal properties.

The plant is native to India and the tropical islands of the Indian Ocean. Besides Madagascar, *Centella asiatica* grows in India, Pakistan, Sri Lanka, Indonesia, East Africa, and South Africa. The leaves of the plant are about the size of an old English penny, which is why the plant is known to English speakers as the pennywort. Its other names are white rot, marsh penny, thick-leaved pennywort, Indian water navelwort, and hydrocotyle. In Sanskrit, *Centella asiatica* is known as *brahmi,* which means "knowledge." In India, the plant is called *gotu kola.* In Madagascar, the plant is called the *talapetraka.*

INTRODUCING *CENTELLA ASIATICA*

Centella asiatica is a slender, herbaceous, ground-hugging plant that thrives in the dark, humid, swampy shadows of the rainforest. Pale pink flowers blossom from the plant from June to September. Extracts are taken from the stalks and rounded leaves. *Centella asiatica* must be harvested in the wilds of the rainforest. Attempts at cultivating *Centella asiatica*

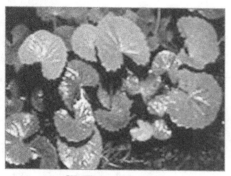

CENTELLA ASIATICA

domestically have failed to produce plants of medicinal value. It seems that *Centella asiatica* needs the stress of its natural environment in order to produce the chemical constituents—asiaticoside, brahmoside, brahminoside, madecassoside, and others—from which its healing power comes.

A Malagasy scientist named Rakoto Ratsimamanga is credited with bringing *Centella asiatica* to the attention of the world. Ratsimamanga knew that the ombiasy, the traditional healers of his native country, use the dried, crushed leaves of *Centella asiatica* to treat leprosy, burns, bronchitis, asthma, and syphilis. In 1956, he conducted an experiment in which patients with chronic skin ulcers were treated with a *Centella asiatica* extract. After three weeks of treatment, ulcers in seventeen of the twenty-two patients were completely healed. Along with another scientist named Boiteau, Ratsimamanga published the results of his experiment in the journal *Thérapie,* and *Centella asiatica* has been the subject of numerous experiments and clinical trials ever since. Two important extracts of the plant, madecassic acid and madecassoside, are named after Madagascar.

Extracts of the plant can be found in hand creams, aftershave lotions, and facial creams, as well as pharmaceutical drugs. *Centella asiatica* stimulates collagen production and, in so doing, restores smoothness to the skin. Pharmaceutical extracts from *Centella asiatica* have proven especially useful in these areas:

- **Tissue development.** *Centella asiatica* helps repair wounds and broken tissue, strengthens cartilage, and heals burns. It also reduces the formation of scar tissue and prevents cellulite from forming.

- **Circulatory and venous problems.** Clinical studies have shown that *Centella asiatica* strengthens the veins and capillaries and improves the flow of blood. Drugs made from the plant are sometimes given to bedridden patients and others who are unable to get exercise or move about. Phlebitis, varicose veins, and inflammation of the veins are also treated with *Centella asiatica* extracts.

Certain animals seem to understand the medicinal value of the plant. The plant is sometimes called "tiger's grass" in India because the Bengal tiger has been known to roll on the plant to heal its wounds after a fight. In Sri Lanka, elephants enjoy dining on *Centella asiatica*—and the elephant, it so happens, has a reputation for longevity. Sri Lankans believe that *Centella asiatica* promotes long life in humans.

The Chemistry of *Centella asiatica*

Centella asiatica contains many substances that aid in wound healing and prevent inflammation. The following triterpenoid compounds in *Centella asiatica* are credited with giving the plant its medicinal value:

- **Asiatic acid.** The compound helps prevent wrinkles and firms the skin. It improves circulation and prevents excessive scar tissue, or keloid, from forming.

- **Asiaticoside.** The compound helps wounds and lesions heal more quickly. It stimulates the formation of fibroblasts, the collagen cells that form a mesh to shape the skin. Asiaticoside also increases blood supply to wounded tissue. It is similar to a steroid in its chemical composition.

- **Madecassic acid.** The compound aids in the synthesis of collagen and tissue regeneration.

- **Madecassoside.** A strong anti-inflammatory agent, it helps blood circulation.

MEDICINAL USES FOR *CENTELLA ASIATICA*

In Ayurveda, the traditional medicine of India, the leaves of *Centella asiatica* are supposed to aid the Crown chakra, the energy center at the top of the head that plays an important role in meditation. Before meditating or practicing yoga, monks drink *Centella asiatica* in a tea to fortify their minds and spirits. *Centella asiatica* is believed to improve the memory and make the person who takes it more articulate. In traditional Indian medicine, *Centella asiatica* is said to bolster the immune system and strengthen the adrenal glands.

In the Far East, traditional healers prescribe the plant to people who suffer from tuberculosis and leprosy, as well as eczema, insect bites, and itching. Modern plastic surgeons have discovered that massaging scar tissue with extracts from *Centella asiatica* helps bring about more acceptable aesthetic results.

Pharmaceutical extracts from *Centella asiatica* have been the subject of nearly fifty years of clinical trials and experiments. It is probably studied more than any essential oil for wound-healing effects. The rest of this chapter highlights clinical experiments that were conducted with *Centella asiatica* extracts.

Centella asiatica and Wound Healing

Collagen is the most abundant protein in the skin. The cells that make collagen are called fibroblasts. Fibroblasts form a gluelike mesh that shapes the skin and gives it its suppleness and flexibility. When you get a cut or scrape, fibroblasts in your skin form the tissue that eventually encloses the wound. Compounds in *Centella asiatica* appear to stimulate the formation of fibroblasts.

In a 1996 study on rats conducted in India, an extract from *Centella asiatica* increased the cellular proliferation and collagen synthesis of wounds. The extract was applied topically. Wounds in rats that did not receive the extract healed significantly more slowly.

In a 1998 study undertaken in India, *Centella asiatica* in ointment, cream, and gel form was applied topically to open wounds in rats. Again, the wounds epithelialized—that is, they closed—more quickly than the wounds in rats that did not receive the extract. The scientists who conducted the experiment reported that the gel formulation worked better than the ointment or cream.

Radiation therapy damages the skin. If the skin is burned too badly, patients may have to postpone further radiation therapy and run the risk of permitting the cancer for which they are being treated to spread. In 1999, scientists in Taiwan irradiated rats and treated the rats' burned skin with a Madécassol extract of *Centella asiatica*. Examining the rats under a microscope, the scientists discovered that the extract had reduced the rats' acute radiation reaction. It had done so, they concluded, by its anti-inflammatory action.

Centella asiatica and Psoriasis

Psoriasis is a major inflammation-associated scaling of the skin, with possible genetic predisposition. As cells on the surface layer of the skin—the keratinocytes—reproduce faster than cells underneath, scales develop. Many scientists believe that psoriasis is the result of an immune system disorder. Normally, T cells protect the body against infection and disease, but a trick of the immune system makes T cells cause inflammation on the skin, and this in turn triggers the cell growth that causes psoriasis. About 6 million Americans suffer from psoriasis. A third of cases are inherited. In a bioassay conducted in London, an aqueous extract of _Centella asiatica_ demonstrated a clear ability to prevent the spread of psoriasis. The researchers concluded that two triterpenoids, madecassoside and asiaticoside, were responsible for the extract's effectiveness.

Centella asiatica and Scleroderma

Scleroderma (the word means "hard skin") is an abnormal thickening of connective tissue of the skin. There may be a link between scleroderma and silicone breast implants, as women with implants appear to be more prone to the disease. About 300,000 people in the United States have scleroderma. Scientists believe that the disease is caused by an autoimmune reaction in which the body overproduces collagen.

In 1998, scientists in Russia undertook a six-month trial in which patients with scleroderma were given the _Centella asiatica_ extract Madécassol. Eighteen patients in the study received the extract in tablet form, forty-two received it as an ointment, and three received it as a powder. After the six-month period, the disease had regressed in twelve patients and not progressed in ten patients. The scientists concluded that Madécassol is effective, especially in topical use—the ointment works better against scleroderma because it is absorbed better.

Centella asiatica, Varicose Veins, and Hemorrhoids

Varicose veins and so-called spider veins are blood vessels that have twisted and swollen. The condition is caused by a leak in a vein's one-way valve or a weakening of the blood vessel wall. By age fifty-five, half of the population has varicose veins. Pregnant women are very susceptible to the condition. The best way to prevent varicose veins is to increase blood circulation to your legs, the part of the body where varicose veins usually appear. You can do that by exercising, keeping your weight down, and wearing comfortable clothing. Hemorrhoids are varicose veins that occur inside the anus and under the skin around the outside of the anus.

Centella asiatica appears to improve microcirculation, capillary flow, and vascular tone. Extracts protect the structure of the blood vessel wall and help new cells grow on blood vessel walls. In so doing, they make the membranes along the blood vessel walls stronger and prevent varicose veins and hemorrhoids from developing.

Centella asiatica and Hypertrophic Scar Tissue

Some racial groups, namely Africans and Asians, are more prone than others to developing hypertrophic scars and keloids. These unsightly scars are shiny and have a pronounced shape. Post-surgery hypertrophic scars and keloids are a problem for millions of people worldwide. In a study conducted in France, a Madécassol extract of *Centella asiatica* was compared to other healing techniques and a placebo drug to see which could do more to prevent post-surgical hypertrophic scars. In the study, the *Centella asiatica* extract was deemed most effective compared to compression bandaging and intralesional cortisone as well as the placebo.

Centella asiatica and Stretch Marks

Extracts from *Centella asiatica* are the only known substances that can prevent stretch marks, or striae, as they are known to the scientific community. These marks appear on the skin when you gain weight quickly or become pregnant. Stretch marks are caused by excess collagen. In effect, the collagen forms scars on the skin as the skin is stretched out of shape. Stretch marks usually appear on the thighs, hips, buttocks, and breasts. They often appear on the skin of adolescents because children grow so quickly during that stage of life.

Knowing the ability of *Centella asiatica* to synthesize collagen, a group at the University of Barcelona undertook a double-blind study to find out whether a *Centella asiatica* extract cream could prevent stretch marks on pregnant women. The extract in the experiment contained asiaticoside as the major active principle. In the placebo group, twenty-two women (56 percent) developed stretch marks, but only fourteen women (34 percent) in the *Centella asiatica* group developed stretch marks. Interestingly, women in the study who developed stretch marks during puberty developed no stretch marks whatsoever when applying the *Centella asiatica* extract during their pregnancy.

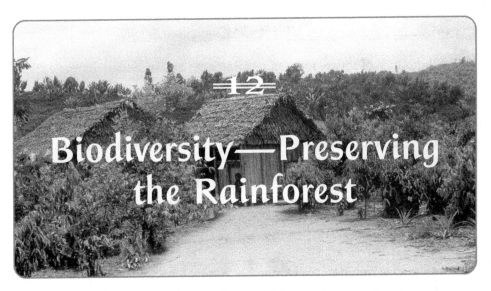

Biodiversity—Preserving the Rainforest

Without the forest, there will be no more water;
without water, there will be no more rice.

—*Malagasy proverb*

The World Wildlife Fund and Conservation International recognize Madagascar as one of the earth's most important "biodiversity hot spots." A biodiversity hot spot is an area where an alarming number of endemic animal and plant species are rapidly losing their habitat. Eight of ten plants found on Madagascar are endemic to the island. Ninety percent of Madagascar's 250 reptile species are endemic. All of its primates are endemic. Wildlife habitats are threatened nearly everywhere in Madagascar.

This chapter examines the problem of how to maintain biodiversity and preserve Madagascar's rainforests. It explains slash-and-burn agricultural techniques and looks into why farmers continue to slash and burn in spite of the damage they do to the rainforest. To demonstrate why preserving the rainforest is important to science and medicine, we tell the story of the Madagascar periwinkle, the little flower that has done so much to ease the suffering of people who have Hodgkin's disease and leukemia.

This chapter looks into two strategies, ecotourism and sustainable agriculture, that may help Madagascar cope with its ecological dilemmas. Along the way, we profile Phael-Flor, an exciting company that is proving why sustainable agriculture offers great opportunities for the island.

MADAGASCAR ON FIRE

Madagascar is on fire. Fires consume about half of the island's savannahs and thousands of square miles of its rainforests and secondary forests each year. In the humid east, smoke plumes rise over the land in the dry months of September, October, and November. The highlands burn in the spring, from August to October. In the drier western region, fires burn from May to November. Most fires are set by cattlemen to clear the land of bush and help the young grass grow. Many fires, however, are set by farmers to clear the land for cultivation. Still more fires result from the frequent use of charcoal, which is the primary source of energy in rural areas.

Writing in *The Eighth Continent,* Peter Tyson describes an airplane ride over Madagascar:

> As soon as you pass over a band of coastal forest, whether rainforest in the east, dry forest in the west, or spiny desert in the south, you enter a barren land. Mile after mile after mile, you see below you bare, treeless hills or plains, often gouged by erosion gullies and blackened by bush fires. On a clear day, this view stretches to the horizon in every direction, and you feel as if you're looking at the surface of another planet—a dead planet. If you come at the end of the dry season, the smoke from these countless fires burning out of control below makes the view even more apocalyptic.

A LOOK AT SLASH-AND-BURN AGRICULTURE

Slash-and-burn farming is an ancient agricultural practice that is now considered harmful to tropical rainforests. The term "slash and burn" was coined rather recently; formerly it was known as "bush-fallowing," "shifting cultivation," and "swidden agriculture." Until the last century, when population pressure made slash-and-burn farming untenable, few people thought to criticize the practice. As long as population densities are low, slash-and-burn farming is an ecologically harmless activity because land that has been slashed and burned, farmed, and abandoned to the forest can lie fallow for long periods of time. The land can be rejuvenated and burned again. When population densities are high, however, land does not remain fallow long enough for the rainforest to rejuvenate it. Farmers have to grow crops on land that is not ready to be farmed—and yields fall accordingly. What's more, farmers come under pressure to slash and burn virgin land.

No one is certain how many people worldwide practice slash-and-burn farming, but estimates range from 240 to 500 million. Nearly half of the land in the tropics has been subject to slashing and burning. Teaching more advanced techniques to the farmers who currently practice slash-and-burn agriculture is difficult. The farmers must learn to use fertilizers and insecticides. They must learn to build drainage systems. Hardest of all, farmers who live from hand to mouth must learn to plan ahead. Switching from slash-and-burn farming to advanced agricultural techniques requires capital that most poor farmers can only dream of.

In the slash-and-burn method, farmers start by clearing the land and letting the cleared vegetation dry. Then the vegetation is either burned or, if it is too wet to burn, left to decompose on its own. In a tropical rainforest, nutrients are stored in plant matter itself, not in the soil (by contrast, the majority of nutrients in a temperate forest are stored in the soil). Burning releases nutrients from plants in the form of ash. The ash serves as a kind of fertilizer. It raises the phosphorus level of the soil and makes the soil less acidic. Typically, farmers can work a slashed-and-burned plot of land for two or three years before the soil is exhausted. Land must remain fallow for ten to twenty years before it can be rejuvenated by the rainforest, burned, and farmed again.

Slashing and burning offers real benefits to farmers. Land can be cleared in a relatively short period of time. The fires drive away rodents and snakes (no small consideration in the tropics). Few implements are needed. Crops can be grown on steep hillsides where plough animals cannot get footing and crops can't normally be grown. Weeding isn't particularly necessary until the second year, when the rainforest begins encroaching on the land. With the forest so close by, birds and other animals act as a kind of natural pesticide and prey on insects that harm the crops.

But slashing and burning is not an efficient farming method in the long term. Due to the lengthy fallow periods that are needed, slash-and-burn farming requires 37 to 74 acres (15 to 30 hectares) per year to feed one person. The soil is soon degraded. Without the forest cover, more rainwater reaches the soil to cause erosion and flush out nutrients. Phosphorus, calcium, magnesium, and potassium are drained from the soil and the soil becomes more acidic. More sunlight reaches the soil, too. The effect is an increase in soil temperature, which retards the formation of humus, the organic portion of the soil that feeds plants. Higher soil temperatures kill healthy microbes and mycorrhizal fungi that contribute to soil health. After a plot of land has been through several slash-and-burn cycles, it must remain fallow for a long period of time, usually sixty years or more, to regain its fertility. In some cases, animal species lose their natural habitats because of slash-and-burn agriculture. Occasionally, fires rage out of control. In 1998, for example, slash-and-burn farmers started a fire in the Amazon state of Roraima that raged for three months and scorched 13,200 square miles before spring rains put it out.

Slash-and-burn farming is not the only threat to the rainforest. Rainforests are disappearing as well under pressure from logging, cattle ranching, and the cutting of timber for fuel. Logging poses an attendant threat to the rainforest. Loggers build roads deep into the forest—roads that farmers can follow to reach remote areas that they could not otherwise reach. Thanks to advances in high-resolution satellite photography, scientists can inventory and track changes to the world's rainforest reserves. By comparing satellite photos taken over a period of years, scientists can observe the effect that logging roads have on deforestation. First come the roads, reaching like river tributaries deeper and deeper into the rainforest. Over time, great swathes of rainforest disappear from the sides of the roads. Eventually the original logging roads cannot be seen in the satellite photographs because so much of the nearby forest has been cut down.

TAVY, SYMBOL OF INDEPENDENCE AND LIBERTY

Often overlooked in discussions about why people in tropical climates engage in slash-and-burn farming is the matter of political oppression. Farms burned into the rainforest are usually found deep in the interior, far from pesky colonial officers, corrupt policemen, undisciplined soldiers, zealous tax collectors, and apparatchiks. The twenty years following the French annexation of Madagascar in 1896 was a period of unrest, famine, and political uncertainty. Some historians point to this period as the beginning of large-scale slashing and burning in Madagascar. Deep in the rainforest, the refugees from French rule engaged in the only economic activity available to them, slash-and-burn rice farming, a practice the Malagasies call *tavy*. According to historian J. Hornac, 70 percent of the primary rainforest in Madagascar was destroyed in the thirty years between 1895 and 1925.

The French agricultural program encouraged farmers to grow coffee beans for the lucrative export market. Fertile land that was previously devoted to rice was given to growing coffee. Rice growers, meanwhile, could not pay the high wages that were being paid on the coffee plantations, and they had trouble getting hands to work their fields. The result was a fall in rice production and widespread hunger. For the first time in memory, the island didn't have enough rice to feed its people. Peasants took to the rainforests to grow food. In larger numbers than before, they engaged in *tavy*, the slashing and burning of the rainforest to produce rice.

In 1909, Governor General Victor Augagneur, concerned by the destruction that *tavy* was causing the rainforest, banned the practice. The governor forbade new land from being slashed and burned without the approval of the government. The government set aside land for rice cultivation, but the land for the most part was unproductive. The Malagasies ignored the ban. They continued practicing slash-and-burn agriculture in the rainforest. Writes Lucy Jarosz, "The ban elevated the practice of *tavy* to a symbol of independence and liberty from colonial rule."

Tavy remained a symbol of independence after colonial rule ended in 1960. Farmers practicing *tavy*, no matter how poor, have the satisfaction of working for themselves and being their own bosses. They enjoy a certain amount of freedom, if only because they live deep in the forest where few people can bother them.

THE MADAGASCAR PERIWINKLE

People often cite the Madagascar periwinkle (*Catharanthus roseus madagascariensis*), also called the rosy periwinkle, as an example of why saving the world's rainforests is so important. Alkaloid extracts from the Madagascar periwinkle have dramatically increased patients' chances of surviving Hodgkin's disease and pediatric leukemia. Previous to the discovery of these extracts, a patient's chances of surviving Hodgkin's disease and pediatric leukemia was one in ten. Today, nine of ten patients survive those diseases.

The Madagascar periwinkle came to the attention of researchers because traditional healers in Madagascar used it to treat high blood pressure, diabetes, asthma, and menstrual problems. In 1954, Dr. Gordon Svoboda, a researcher at Eli Lilly Pharmaceuticals in Switzerland, discovered that two alkaloids in the leaves of the plant, vincristine and vinblastine, could slow the progress of leukemia. In the 1960s, Eli Lilly introduced two anticancer drugs derived from the Madagascar periwinkle. Vincristine is used to treat pediatric leukemia and vinblastine to treat Hodgkin's disease. These drugs work by impeding the growth of abnormal cancer cells.

Vendors selling medicinal plants and herbs can be found in the outdoor markets of nearly every city and town in Madagascar. In the countryside, ombiasy, the traditional healers, dispense cures in the form of teas, plants, and herbs. The skin of the *kily* (*Tamarindus indica*), for example, is used to treat rheumatism and measles. The leaves of the *voafotsy* (*Aploia theaeformis*) are taken for malaria. One wonders how many of these traditional plant cures could be useful to modern medicine. According to the International Wildlife Federation, only 1 percent of the world's rainforest plant species has been tested for medical use. One wonders as well how many healing plants in Madagascar are lost forever as the rainforests are consumed by fire.

ECOTOURISM AS A CONSERVATION STRATEGY

Many Malagasies have pinned their hopes on ecotourism as a way to preserve the ecological diversity of Madagascar and provide people with a means of livelihood. Ecotourism is the fastest growing segment of the $3.5 trillion travel industry. Madagascar has much to offer the ecotourist in terms of exotic wildlife and natural beauty. The island's thirty-six national parks and nature reserves, which comprise 1.8 percent of the land, are an ideal destination for tourists who enjoy viewing wildlife and experiencing natural habitats firsthand.

In 1980, the government embarked on an ambitious program to maintain the nation's parks and wildlife areas and create new reserves as well. With the help of the World Wildlife Fund for Nature (WWF), programs educating students in the importance of ecology were introduced in the schools. In the 1990s, the program was modified to make participation by the people who live near the parks and wildlife areas a goal. Programs in which revenues from parks and reserves are shared with local villagers have been set up across Madagascar with the help of the United States Agency for International Development (USAID).

Malagasies who promote ecotourism point to Costa Rica, another country with rainforest reserves and exotic wildlife, as a model for what Madagascar could become. Ecotourism is now the primary source of revenue in Costa Rica. Madagascar, however, is many times larger than Costa Rica. Traveling in Madagascar is much more difficult. Accommodations for tourists are more primitive. And Madagascar is far from Europe and North America, where the majority of ecotourists make their homes. As well as preserving land, the government has to allocate resources for building roads and upgrading the infrastructure before ecotourism becomes a viable source of income for Madagascar.

PRACTICING SUSTAINABLE AGRICULTURE WITH PHAEL-FLOR

The other strategy for preserving Madagascar's biodiversity is sustainable agriculture. Sustainability is based on the principle that meeting the needs of the present should not compromise future generations' ability to meet their needs. In Madagascar, sustainable agriculture means earning a living from the land without destroying the rainforest.

In the countryside near Moramanga, about 100 kilometers (62 miles) east of Antananarivo, an innovative company called Phael-Flor is demonstrating that sustainable agriculture is profitable as well as possible in Madagascar. The company was formed in 1981 by Rolland Ramboatiana, a French-educated chemist and biologist (he named the company after his parents, Raphael and Flora). The company was formed to cultivate aromatic and medicinal plants and manufacture essential oils. Extraction of essential oils is done at the company's 100-acre facility in the countryside. Phael-Flor may well be the only essential oil producer on the island that distills oil on site. The company's overriding philosophy is to strive for environmental health, as well as economic profitability.

Phael-Flor cultivates geranium, ravintsara, lemongrass, ginger, citronella, sweet basil, and vetiver. The company has provided an economic boost to the nearby villagers who are either employed by the company or sell it items it needs, such as manure and foodstuffs. Villagers have learned how to cultivate the plants and distill essential oils. Instead of cutting down wood to fuel the distillation, Phael-Flor purchases wood scraps from a nearby mill.

The company actively participates in the region's social development by donating money to local schools. Phael-Flor is planning to build a small health clinic so that workers don't have to walk the 10 kilometers (6.2 miles) to Moramanga for health services. The poorest workers are lodged without charge in prefab wooden houses that the company provides.

Phael-Flor has been able to cut production costs and increase its profits by producing essential oil on site. Because the company doesn't have to truck ginger to a distillery, it can make essential oil from fresh ginger without having to dry it. Phael-Flor's essential oil from fresh ginger has won praise in Europe. The oil is more faithful to the plant. It is spicier, stronger, more volatile, and fresher than conventional ginger oil. It doesn't have conventional ginger's dry, woodsy smell. Ramboatiana credits his company's unique ginger oil to the presence of sesquiterpenes, which are normally lost during drying. Very few companies produce ginger essential oil from fresh ginger, but Phael-Flor can do it because it has set up its operations in the countryside.

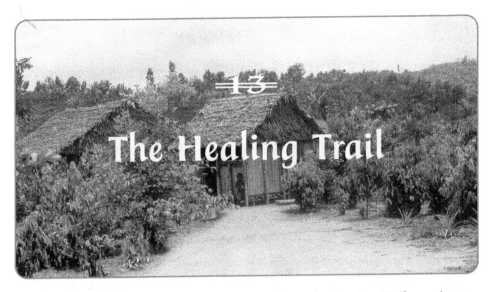

The Healing Trail

T his book gets its title and inspiration from the Healing Trail, a unique tour of Madagascar designed especially for aromatherapists, massage practitioners, and health-care providers who use essential oils in their work. The eco-tour was designed by Roger Rakotomalala, a native of Madagascar, for his San Francisco-based company, Lemur Tours. The idea behind the Healing Trail is to introduce aromatherapists and other interested parties to the essential oils of Madagascar and the people who make them. Along the way, tourists immerse themselves in the country and come away with an experience more intense and heartfelt than they would otherwise have had.

"The Healing Trail is a way for tourists to truly discover Madagascar," says Rakotomalala. "The island is known for its nature and wildlife, and the tour gives people plenty of opportunities to see that. But because it focuses on essential oils and how they are made, it gives tourists an entrée into the culture. Visitors get closer to the people who make essential oils. Of course, they also have a great time exploring the rainforests, snorkeling, and doing the other traditional tourist things."

The tour is a blend of the recreational and the educational. Always accompanied by an English-speaking guide, tourists trek into the rainforest to observe and breathe in the fragrance of the wild ravintsara tree, the cinnamon tree, the foraha tree, and other plants from which essential oils are made. Visitors hear lectures by authorities in the field of botany and essential oil production, as well. They get the opportunity to talk to local healers and find out how the Malagasies use medicinal plants and herbs. They see firsthand how plants are cultivated, harvested, and distilled into essential oils. On the Healing Trail, visitors learn how to educate themselves in what makes a good essential oil and how to identify high-quality oils.

The Healing Trail is in many ways like aromatherapy itself. As visitors encounter essential oils and healing plants, they awaken to the sights, smells, and sounds of Madagascar—and they experience the island on a deeper, more personal level.

The tour is not, however, only about essential oils. The Healing Trail also offers all the traditional, classic tourist experiences of Madagascar. Visitors can explore the Perinet reserve at dawn as mist rises from the rainforest canopy, hunt for wild orchids, take a leisurely trip on the Pangalanes canal, explore the outdoor markets, photograph the sacred black lemurs of Nosy Kamba, or even swim in the warm tropical waters of Nosy Tanikely.

Although the tour takes visitors deep into the countryside where they would not otherwise go, Rakotomalala goes out of his way to provide his guests with comfortable accommodations. One of the goals of the tour is to introduce aromatherapists to one another, and Rakotomalala wanted a relaxed setting where aromatherapists could trade ideas and experiences at the end of the day. Healing Trail tourists being who they are, they sometimes enhance their experience by giving one another massages with Malagasy essential oils—and participation is officially encouraged.

The Healing Trail is an extraordinary tour of Madagascar that has been richly flavored and enlivened by the country's essential oils. Anyone interested in taking the tour may contact tour guide Roger Rakotomalala at this address:

Lemur Tours, Inc.
501 Mendell Street, #B
San Francisco, CA 94124
Tel: 1-800-73LEMUR • Fax: 415-695-8899
www.lemurtours.com

APPENDIX A

Obtaining Essential Oils from Madagascar

We recommend purchasing essential oils from Madagascar from the company listed here:

Lemur 2000 Inc.–Phael-Flor USA
 501 Mendell Street, #B
 San Francisco, CA 94124
 Tel: 1-800-73LEMUR or 415-695-8880
 Fax: 415-695-8899 • E-mail: LemurInc@aol.com

Lemur 2000 Inc.–Phael-Flor USA offers the following essential oils and herbs:

NAME	AVAILABILITY	CERTIFICATION
Black pepper (*Piper nigrum*)	Starting in June	Pending
Cinnamon bark (*Cinnamomum zeylanicum*)	All year	Eco-certified
Cinnamon leaf (*Cinnamomum zeylanicum*)	All year	Eco-certified
Clove bud (*Eugenia caryophyllata*)	November through March	Eco-certified
Combava	All year	Wild-crafted
Foraha oil (*Calophyllum inophyllum*)	All year	Wild-crafted
Geranium leaf (*Pelargonium roseum*)	Starting in March, 3 times per year	Eco-certified
Ginger root (*Zingiber officinale*)	May through September	Eco-certified

NAME	AVAILABILITY	CERTIFICATION
Green pepper (*Piper nigrum*)	March through May	Pending
Havozo (*Ravintsara anisata*)	All year	Eco-certified
Katrafay (*Cedrelopsis grevel*)	All year	Pending
Niaouli (*Melaleuca viridiflora*)	All year	Eco-certified
Pine (*Pinus kessia*)	All year	Eco-certified
Radriaka (*Lantana camara*)	February through March	Eco-certified
Ravintsara leaf (*Ravensara aromatica*)	All year	Eco-certified
Tagete (*Tagete bipinata*)	February through April	Wild-crafted
Vanilla absolute (*Vanilla planifolia*)	All year	Eco-certified
Wild orange petit grains (*Citrus aurantifolia*)	All year	Pending
Ylang-ylang (*Canaga odorata*) Complete	November through March	Eco-certified
Ylang-ylang (*Canaga odorata*) Grade 3	November through March	Eco-certified

Traveling to Madagascar

Madagascar's great luxury is space, luminous,
beautiful emptiness, mile after mile of grassland,
brush, and woodland, broken by craggy mountains.

—Arthur Stratton, *The Great Red Island*

If you are looking for the unexpected and you want to meet extraordinary people, Madagascar is the place to go. "Apart from the Tibetans," wrote travel writer Dervla Murphy in *Muddling Through in Madagascar*, "I have never traveled among a people as endearing as the Malagasy."

GETTING THE HELP OF TRAVEL PROFESSIONALS

We recommend getting the help of a travel professional as you plan your trip to Madagascar. Tourism is a young industry on the island. The roads are not the best, especially in the rainy season. Madagascar is vast. The Malagasy language can be daunting. Traveling from place to place and finding accommodations isn't easy. A travel professional can help you choose where to travel on the island and chart your course from place to place.

If you have plenty of time for your trip and you are extremely patient, you can go it on your own. But you will spend an inordinate amount of time finding out how to get from destination to destination when you could be on the move already with the help of a travel professional.

The U.S. State Department maintains a travel advisory about Madagascar at these Web sites: www.travel.state.gov/madagascar.html and www.state.gov/p/af/ci/ma.

TRAVEL COSTS

Contrary to conventional wisdom, traveling in Madagascar is not cheap. Traveling to and from the island from North America costs about $2,000. After you arrive, expect to spend about $150 per day for hotel accommodations, meals, and shopping. Madagascar has almost no industries. Most building materials and fuel have to be imported. To live in conditions similar to what you are accustomed to at home, you have to pay high prices.

The Malagasy currency is called the Malagasy franc or *Franc Malgache* (FMG). As of October 2002, one American dollar buys 6,712 FMG; one euro buys 6,577 FMG. Money can be changed at banks, airports, and some hotels. Credit cards are slowly gaining acceptance and can be used in major cities.

OBTAINING A VISA

A visa is required for traveling in Madagascar. To obtain a visa, you must get an application form from the embassy or one of the consulates or missions listed below. Fill out the application and return it. You can do so by mail.

The cost of the visa is $33 to $39, depending on how long you want to stay. Everyone who applies for a visa must provide the following:

• A valid passport
• Passport photograph
• Completed application form
• Copy of a round-trip ticket or itinerary

Travelers who wish to stay longer than three months must obtain a business visa.

Embassy of the Republic of Madagascar
2374 Massachusetts Avenue N.W.
Washington, DC 20008
Tel: 202-265-5525
Fax: 202-265-3034
www.embassy.org/madagascar

Honorary Consulate of Madagascar
1318 Santa Luisa Drive
Solana Beach, CA 92075
Tel: 858-792-6999
Fax: 858-792-5280
E-mail: info@madagascar-consulate.org
www.madagascar-consulate.org

Honorary Consulate of Madagascar
2299 Piedmont Avenue
Berkeley, CA 94720
Tel: 510-643-8301
Fax: 510-643-3993
E-mail:
lkozial@uclink.berkeley.edu

Honorary Consulate of Madagascar
123 South Broad Street
Philadelphia, PA 19109
Tel: 215-893-3067

Mission of Madagascar at the United Nations
820 Second Avenue, Suite 800
New York, NY 10017
Tel: 212-744-3816

Embassy of Madagascar
649 Vlair Road
Ottawa, ON K1J 7M4
Canada
Tel: 613-744-7995
Fax: 613-744-2530

Honorary Consulate of Madagascar
69-7C Mark Lane
London EC3 R75A
England
Tel: 44-171-480-3899

ENTRY REQUIREMENTS

Besides a valid visa and passport, evidence of yellow fever and/or cholera immunization is required for travelers who have been in an infected zone in the six months previous to their arrival in Madagascar.

Health Requirements

Malaria is a problem in the lowland coastal areas of Madagascar. Consult your health-care provider four to eight weeks before leaving to find out which antimalarial drug to take, given your travel itinerary. Some doctors recommend vaccinations for hepatitis A, typhoid fever, and polio for visitors to Madagascar.

WHEN TO TRAVEL

The best time to travel to Madagascar is April to October, when the weather is cooler and drier. The rainy season lasts from November to March. Madagascar, however, is huge, and temperatures and rainfall vary from region to region.

HOW TO GET THERE

Direct flights to Madagascar are not available from the United States or Canada. Flights depart from London, Paris, Geneva, Frankfurt, Rome, and Zurich for Antananarivo, the capital of Madagascar. You can also fly to Madagascar from Réunion Island and Mauritius.

Notes

Chapter 1

Brown, M., *Madagascar Rediscovered: A History From Early Times To Independence*, Hamden, CT: Archon Books 1979.

Burney, D.A., et al., The *kilopilopitsofy, kidoky,* and *bokyboky:* accounts of strange animals from Belo-Sur-Mer, Madagascar, and the megafaunal "extinction window," *American Anthropologist,* 100: 4, 957–966, 1998.

Chalot, C., La culture des plantes à parfums dans les colonies françaises, *Agronomie Coloniale,* 112: 105, 1927.

Deschamps, H.J., *Madagascar,* Paris, France: Presses Universitaires de France, 1968.

Diamond, J., *Guns, Germs, and Steel: The Fates of Human Societies,* New York: W.W. Norton & Co., 1999.

Diamond, S., Beauty in peril: the stoltmann wilderness, *HerbalGram,* 48: 50–62, 2000.

Duke, J.A., *Handbook of Medicinal Herbs,* Boca Raton, FL: CRC Press, 1985.

Frazer, J.G., *The Native Races of Africa and Madagascar: A Copious Selection of Passages for The Study of Social Anthropology From The Manuscript Notebooks of Sir James George Frazier,* Downie, R.A., ed., New York: AMS Press, 1975.

Kent, R.K., *From Madagascar to the Malagasy Republic.* New York: Praeger, 1962.

Kouwenhoven, A.P., *Madagascar: The Red Island.* Leiden, Holland: WINCO Publishing, 1995.

Lyautey, L.H.G., *Lettres Du Sud De Madagascar, 1900–1902. Avec Un Portrait et Une Carte Hors Texte,* Paris, France: A Colin, 1935.

Marden, L., Madagascar: island at the end of the earth, *National Geographic,* 132: 4, 443–487, October 1967.

Mauro, D., *Madagascar l'Ile essentielle,* Paris, France: Emeline Raholiarisoa Anako, 2000.

Osborn, C.S., *Madagascar. Land of the Man-Eating Tree,* New York: Republic Publishing Company, 1924.

Powell, E.A., *Beyond the Utmost Purple Rim: Abyssinia, Somaliland, Kenya Colony, Zanzibar, The Comoros, and Madagascar,* New York: The Century Co., 1925.

Preston-Mafham, K., *Madagascar: A Natural History,* New York: Facts on File, 1991.

Rakotoarisoa, J., A cultural history of Madagascar: evolution and interpretation of the archaeological evidence, In *Natural Change and Human Impact in Madagascar.* Goodman, S., et al., eds., Washington, DC: Smithsonian Institution Press, 1997.

Rasoanaivo, P., et al., Essential oils of economic value in Madagascar: present state of knowledge, *HerbalGram,* 43: 31–39, 58–59, 1998.

Richard, J., *Lights And Shadows Or Chequered Experiences Among Some Of The Heathen Tribes of Madagascar,* Antananarivo, Madagascar: London Missionary Society Press, 1877.

Rogozinski, J., *Honor Among Thieves: Caption Kidd, Henry Every, And The Pirate Democracy In The Indian Ocean,* Mechanicsburg, PA: Stackpole Books, 2000.

Sclater, P.L., Mammals of Madagascar, *Quarterly Journal of Science,* 213–219, April 1864.

Secord, A.R., *Robert Drury's Journal And Other Studies,* Urbana, IL: University of Illinois Press 1961.

Stratton, A., *The Great Red Island,* New York: Charles Scribner and Sons, 1964.

Thomas, H., *The Slave Trade: The History Of The Atlantic Slave Trade 1440–1870,* New York: Picador Macmillan, 1997.

Thompsen, V.M., *The Malagasy Republic: Madagascar Today,* Stanford, CA: Stanford University Press, 1965.

Tyson, P., *The Eighth Continent: Life, Death, And Discovery In The Lost World Of Madagascar,* New York: HarperCollins, 2000.

Wallerstein, I., *Africa: The Politics Of Independence,* New York: Random House, 1961.

Wetmore, A., Re-creating Madagascar's giant extinct bird, *National Geographic,* 132:4: 488–493, October 1967.

Wright, H., et al., Cultural transformations and their impacts on the environments of Madagascar, In *Natural Change and Human Impact in Madagascar,* Goodman, S., et al., eds.,Washington, DC: Smithsonian Institution Press, 1997.

Zatkin, S., Help the land of the lemurs move forward, *The Nation.* www.csmonitor.com/2002/0222/p11s03-coop.html, February 22, 2002.

Chapter 2

Bowling, A., *Research Methods In Health,* Buckingham, England: Open University Press, 1997.

Clark, P.E., et al., Therapeutic touch: is there a scientific basis for the practice? *Nursing Research,* 31(3): 37–41, 1984.

Dinar, J., Aromatherapy diffuses sweet smell of success, *Natural Foods Merchandiser,* 34: 17–19, November 2000.

Earle, L., *Vital Oils,* London: Vermillion, 1994.

Farbman, A.I., *Cell Biology Of Olfaction,* Cambridge, England: Cambridge University Press, 1992.

Farkas, A., *Perfume Thru The Ages,* New York: Psychological Library, 1951.

Fischer-Rizzi, S., *Complete Aromatherapy Handbook,* London: Sterling Publishing Co., 1989.

Gobel, H., et al., Effect of peppermint and eucalyptus oil preparations on neurophysiological and experimental algesimetric headache parameters, *Cephalagia* 14: 228–34, 1994.

Hardy, M., et al., Replacement of drug treatment for insomnia by ambient odor (letter), *Lancet,* 346: 701, 1995.

Keville, K., et al., *Aromatherapy: A Complete Guide To The Healing Art,* Santa Cruz, CA: The Crossing Press, 1995.

Kodis, M., et al., *Love Scents: How Your Natural Pheromones Influence Your Relationships, Your Moods, And Who You Love.* New York: Dutton Books, 1998.

Lawless, J., *Aromatherapy And The Mind: The Psychological And Emotional Effects Of Essential Oils.* Wellingborough, England: Thorsons, 1994.

Metcalfe, J., *Herbs And Aromatherapy,* London: Devon, Webb & Bower, Ltd., 1989.

Price, S., et al., *Aromatherapy For Health Professionals,* Edinburgh, Scotland: Churchill Livingstone, 1995.

Proust, M., *A La Recherche Du Temps Perdu,* Paris: Gallimard, 1954.

Rose, J., *The Aromatherapy Book,* Berkeley, CA: North Atlantic Books, 1992.

Ryman, D., *Aromatherapy: The Encyclopedia Of Plants And Oils And How They Help You*, London: Judy Piatkus Publishers, Ltd., 1991.

Schlosser, E., Why McDonald's fries taste so good, *Atlantic Monthly*, 287:50–56, 2001.

Steele, J., et al., Brain research and essential oils, *Aromatherapy Quarterly*, 5, Spring 1984.

Tisserand, R., *The Art Of Aromatherapy*, London: C.W. Daniel Co. Ltd., 1994.

Chapter 3

Armstrong, W., Seed voyagers, *Pacific Discovery*, 43:32–39, 1990.

Cox, P., et al., *Islands, Plants And Polynesians*, Portland, OR: Dioscorides Press, 1991.

Darwin, C., *The Collected Papers Of Charles Darwin*, Vol. 1. Ed. P. Barret. Chicago: University of Chicago Press, 1977.

Gorman, M.L., *Outline Studies In Ecology: Island Ecology*, London: Chapman and Hall, 1979.

Gunn, C., et al., *World Guide To Tropical Drift Seeds And Fruits*, New York: Quadrangle/New York Times Book Co., 1976.

Itoigawa, M., et al., Cancer chemopreventative agents, 4-phenylcoumarins from *calophyllum inophyllum*, *Cancer Lett.*, 169: 15–19, 2001.

Kilham, C., Oil of tamanu profuse in Polynesia, *Natural Foods Merchandiser*, http://nfm-online/nfm_backs/Feb_01/tamanu.cfm, 2001.

Palmer, C., et al., Part 2: synthesis of the *calophyllum coumarins*, *J. Chem. Soc. Perkin. Trans.*, 1: 3135–3152, 1995.

Rasoanaivo, P., et al., Essential oils of economic value in Madagascar: present state of knowledge, *HerbalGram*, 43: 31–39, 58–59, 1998.

Riff, A., From the jungle to the clinic, *Far Eastern Economic Review*, June 14, 2001.

Spino, C., et al., Anti-HIV coumarins from *calophyllum* seed oil, *Bioorg. Med. Chem. Lett.*, 8: 3475–3478, 1998.

Chapter 4

Black, J., E-mail exchange regarding the cineol content of the ravintsara leaf, April 17, 2002.

de Medici, D., et al., Chemical analysis of essential oil of Malagasy medicinal plants by gas chromatography and NMR spectroscopy, *Flav. Fragr. J.*, 7: 275–281, 1992.

Decary, R., Quelques plantes aromatiques et à parfum de la flore de Madagascar, *Journal d'Agriculture Tropicale et de Botanique Appliquées*, 2: 416, 1955.

Groebel, A., et al., Uber die inhaltsstoffe aus *ravensara aromatica* einer auf Madagaskar vorkommenden Lauraceae, *Planta Med.*, 18: 66, 1986.

Mollenbeck, S., et al., Chemical composition and analyses of enantiomers of essential oils from Madagascar, *Flav. Fragr. J.*, 12: 63–69, 1997.

Raharivelomanana, P.J., et al., Study of the antimicrobial action of various essential oils extracted from Malagasy plants. II: Lauraceae, *Arch. Inst. Pasteur. Madagascar*, 56(1): 261–271, 1989.

Rasoanaivo, P., et al., Essential oils of economic value in Madagascar: present state of knowledge, *HerbalGram*, 43: 31–39, 58–59, 1998.

Théron, E., et al., Authentication of *ravensara aromatica* and *ravensara anisata*, *Planta Med.*, 60: 489–491, 1994.

Chapter 5

Akhmadieva, A., et al., The protective action of a natural preparation of anthocyan (pelargonidin-3,5-diglucoside), *Radiobiologia*, 33(3): 433–435, 1993.

Blunt, W., *The Complete Naturalist: A Life Of Linnaeus*, Princeton, NJ: Princeton University Press, 1971.

Clark, D., *Pelargoniums: Kew Gardening Guides*, Portland, OR: Timber Press, 1988.

Earle, L., *Vital Oils*, London: Vermillion, 1994.

Gerard, J., *The Herball Or Generall Historie Of Plants*, Amsterdam: Theatrum Orbis Terrarum, Ltd., 1974 (first published 1633).

Gould, S., *Dinosaur In A Haystack: Reflections In Natural History*, New York: Harmony Books, 1996.

Lavabre, M., *Aromatherapy Workbook*, Montpelier, VT: Healing Arts Press, 1990.

Lawless, J., *Aromatherapy And The Mind: The Psychological And Emotional Effects Of Essential Oils*, Wellingborough, England: Thorsons, 1994.

Lis-Balchin, M., E-mail exchange regarding the *Pelargonium roseum* hybrid, April 16, 2002.

Rasoanaivo, P., et al., Essential oils of economic value in Madagascar: present state of knowledge, *HerbalGram* 43: 31–39, 58–59, 1998.

Rose, J., *The Aromatherapy Book*, Berkeley, CA: North Atlantic Books, 1992.

Ryman, D., *The Aromatherapy Handbook: The Secret Healing Power Of Essential Oils*, London: Piatkus, 1989.

————, *Aromatherapy: The Encyclopedia Of Plants And Oils And How They Help You*, London: Judy Piatkus Publishers, Ltd., 1991.

Yeo, P., *Hardy Geraniums*, Portland, OR: Timber Press, 1985.

Chapter 6

Anthony, A., et al., Metabolism of estragole in rat and mouse and influence of dose size on excretion of the proximate carcinogen 1'-hydroxyestragole, *Food Chem. Toxicol.*, 25: 799–806, 1987.

Bianchi, L.A., et al., Genotoxicity assessment of essential oils extracted from *artemisia draconculus* and *ocimum basilicum* tested in *saccharomyces cerevisiae* D7, *Mutat. Res.*, 216: 298, 1989.

Castleman, M., *The Healing Herbs: The Ultimate Guide To The Curative Power Of Nature's Medicines*, Emmaus, PA: Rodale Press, 1991.

Culpeper, N., *Culpeper's Complete Herbal And English Physician*, Glenwood, IL: Meyerbooks, 1987 (first published in 1652).

Das, S., Tulsi: the holy power plant, *About Us*, http://hinduism.about.com, 2002.

Drinkwater, N., et al., Hepatocarcinogenicity of estragole (1-allyl-4-methoxybenzene) and 1'-hydroxyestragole in the mouse and mutagenicity of 1'-acetoxyestragole in bacteria, *J. Natl. Cancer Inst.*, 57(6): 1323–1331, 1976.

Earle, L., *Vital Oils*. London: Vermillion, 1994.

Elgayyar, M., et al., Antimicrobial activity of essential oils from plants against selected pathogenic and saprophytic microorganisms, *J. Food Prot.*, 64: 1019–1024, 2001.

Giron, L. M., et al., Ethnobotanical survey of the medicinal flora used by the Caribs of Guatemala, *J. Ethnopharmacol*, 34(2–3): 173–187, 1991.

Graedon, J., et al., *The People's Pharmacy: Guide To Home And Herbal Remedies*, New York: St. Martin's Press, 1999.

Hurly, J.B., *The Good Herb: Recipes And Remedies From Nature*, New York: William Morrow and Company, 1995.

Lachowicz, K., et al., The synergistic preservative effects of the essential oils of sweet basil (*ocimum basilicum*) against acid-tolerant food microflora, *Lett. Appl. Microbiol.* 26: 209–214, 1998.

Lawless, J., *Aromatherapy And The Mind: The Psychological And Emotional Effects Of Essential Oils*, London: Thorsons, 1994.

Opinion of the scientific committee on food on estragole (1-Allyl-4-methoxy-benzene), Publication of the European Commission, Health & Consumer Protection Directorate-General, *SCF/CS/Flav/Flavour/6 Add2 Final*, September 26, 2001.

Randriamiharisoa, R.P., et al., Etude de la variation de la composition chimique et classification des huiles essentielles de basilic de Madagascar, *Sciences des Aliments*. 6: 221, 1986.

Rasoanaivo, P., et al., Essential oils of economic value in Madagascar: present state of knowledge, *HerbalGram*, 43: 31–39, 58–59, 1998.

Simon, J.E., et al., Basil: a source of essential oils, In *Advances in New Crops*, Janick, J., et al., eds., 484–489. Portland, OR: Timber Press, 1990.

Tisserand, R., *Essential Oil Safety: A Guide For Health Care Professionals*, London: Churchill Livingstone, 1999.

Wan, J., et al., The effect of essential oils of basil on the growth of *aeromonas hydrophila* and *pseudomonas fluorescens*, *J. Appl. Microbiol.*, 84: 152–158, 1998.

Chapter 7

Chang, S.T., Antibacterial activity of leaf essential oils and their constituents from *cinnamomum osmophloeum*, *J. Ethnopharmacol*, 77(1): 123–127, 2001.

Dalby, A., *Dangerous Tastes: The Story Of Spices*, Los Angeles: University of California Press, 2000.

Dhuley, J.N., Anti-oxidant effects of cinnamon (*cinnamomum verum*) bark and greater cardamom (*amomum subulatum*) seeds in rats fed a high-fat diet, *Indian J. Exp. Biol.*, 37(3): 238–242, 1999.

Gago-Dominguez, M., et al., Lipid peroxidation: a novel and unifying concept of the etiology of renal cell carcinoma, *Cancer—Causes & Control*, 13(3): 287–293, 2002.

Graedon, J., et al., *The People's Pharmacy: Guide To Home And Herbal Remedies*, New York: St. Martin's Press, 1999.

Hughes, M.S., *Flavor Foods: Spices & Herbs. Plants We Eat*, Minneapolis, MN: Lerner Publications Company, 2000.

Jarvill-Taylor, K.J., et al., A hydroxychalcone derived from cinnamon functions as a mimetic for insulin in 3T3-L1 adipocytes, *Am. Coll. Nutr.*, 20(4): 327–336, 2001.

Kern, M.E., et al., *Medical Mycology: A Self-Instructional Text,* Philadelphia: F. A. Davis Co., 1997.

Keville, K., et al., *Aromatherapy: A Complete Guide To The Healing Art,* Santa Cruz, CA: The Crossing Press, 1995.

Khan, A., et al., Insulin potentiating factor and chromium content of selected foods and spices, *Biol. Trace Elem. Res.,* 24(3): 183–188, 1990.

Lawless, J., *Aromatherapy And The Mind: The Psychological And Emotional Effects Of Essential Oils,* London: Thorsons, 1994.

Mancini-Filho, J., et al., Antioxidant activity of cinnamon (*cinnamomum zeylanicum,* breyne) extracts, *Boll Chim. Farm.,* 137(11): 443–447, 1998.

Mau, J., et al., Antimicrobial effect of extracts from Chinese chive, cinnamon, and corni fructus, *J. Agric. Food Chem.* 49(1): 183–188, 2001.

Mayanagi, M., The names of drugs in the cassia-bark family in China prior to the 11th century: on the standardization as Guizhi by Ling Yi and other scholars of cassia-bark family drug names appearing in the medical work by Zhongjing, *Yakushigaku Zasshi,* 30(2): 96–115, 1995.

Miller, J.I., *The Spice Trade Of The Roman Empire, 29 B.C. to 641 A.D.,* Oxford, England: Oxford University Press, 1969.

Morozumi, S., Isolation, purification, and antibiotic activity of o-methoxycinnamaldehyde from cinnamon, *Appl. Environ. Microbiol.,* 36(4): 577–583, 1978.

Nagai, H., et al., Immunopharmacological studies of the aqueous extract of *cinnamomum cassia,* Jpn. *J. Pharmacol.,* 32(5): 813–822, 1982.

Purseglove, J.W., et al., *Spices,* Vol. 1. Tropical Agriculture. New York: Longman Group Ltd., 1981.

Quale, J.M., et al., *In vitro* activity of *Cinnamomum zeylanicum* against azole-resistant and sensitive candida species and a pilot study of cinnamon for oral candidiasis, *Am. J. Chin. Med.,* 24(2): 103–109, 1996.

Raharivelomanana, P.J., Contribution à l'étude des huiles essentielles de Laurus nobilis, *cinnamomum zeylanicum, ravensara anisata* (Lauraceae): composition chimique, inhibition microbienne. Mémoire de DEA, Faculté des Sciences, Université d'Antananarivo, 1988.

Raharivelomanana, P.J., et al., Study of the antimicrobial action of various essential oil extracts from Madagascan plants. II. The Lauraceae. *Archives of the Institute of Pasteur Madagascar.* 56: 261–271, 1989.

Randriamanantena, A.A., Approche technico-économique de l'extraction industrielle d'huile essentielle d'écorces de cannelle. Mémoire de fin d'Etude d'Ingéniorat, Ecole Supérieure des Sciences Agronomiques, Université d'Antananarivo, 1992.

Rasoanaivo, P., et al., Essential oils of economic value in Madagascar: present state of knowledge, *HerbalGram*, 43: 31–39,58–59, 1998.

Razafindramiarana, H., Contribution à l'étude de l'huile essentielle de la canelle. Mémoire de fin d'étude d'Ingéniorat, Ecole Supérieure Agronomique, Université d'Antananarivo, 1985.

Rose, J., *The Aromatherapy Book*, Berkeley, CA: North Atlantic Books, 1992.

Saeki, Y., et al., Antimicrobial action of natural substances on oral bacteria. *Bull. Tokyo Dent. Coll.*, 30(3): 129–135, 1989.

Singh, H.B., et al., Cinnamon bark oil, a potent fungitoxicant against fungi-causing respiratory tract mycoses, *Allergy*, 50(12): 995–999, 1995.

Stuckey, M., *The Complete Spice Book*, New York: St. Martin's Press, 1997.

Tabak, M., et al., Cinnamon extracts' inhibitory effect on *Helicobacter pylori*, *J. Ethnopharmacol.*, 67(3): 269–277, 1999.

Underriner, E.W., et al., *Handbook Of Industrial Seasonings*, London: Blackie Academic & Professional, 1994.

Veal, L., The potential effectiveness of essential oils as a treatment for head lice (*Pediculus humanus capitis*), *Complement. Ther. Nurs. Midwifery*, 2(4): 97–101, 1996.

Vogono, F., et al., Contribution à l'étude de quelques huiles essentielles, concrètes et absolues de plantes aromatiques de Madagascar, Mémoire de fin d'Etude d'Ingéniorat, Ecole Supérieure Polytechnique, Université d'Antananarivo, 1987.

Waijesekera, R.O., Historical overview of the cinnamon industry. *CRC Crit. Rev. Food Sci. Nutri.*, 10(1): 1–30, 1978.

Wild, A., *The East India Company Book Of Spices*. London: Harper Collins, 1995.

Zhang, Z., et al., Comparison of bacteriostatic ability of oleum of *perfilla frutescens* (L.) Britt., *cinnamomum cassia* Presl and Nipagin A, *Zhongguo Zhong Yao Za Zhi*, 15(2): 95–97, 126–127, 1990.

Chapter 8

Bartley, J.P., et al., Supercritical extraction of Australian grown ginger, *J. Sci. Food Agri.*, 66: 365, 1994.

Carr, I., Folk healing, alternative, and parallel medicines, *Neil John Maclean*

Health Sciences Library, http://www.umanitoba.ca/.../histories/folk.html, 1997.

Castleman, M., *The Healing Herbs: The Ultimate Guide To The Curative Power Of Nature's Medicines,* Emmaus, PA: Rodale Press, 1991.

Chang, K.C., ed., *Food In Chinese Culture,* New Haven, CT: Yale University Press, 1977.

Denyer, C.V., et al., Isolation of antirhinoviral sesquiterpenes from ginger. *J. Nat. Prod.,* 57(5): 658–662, 1004.

Earle, L., *Vital Oils,* London: Vermillion, 1994.

Fuler, S., *The Ginger Book: The Ultimate Home Remedy,* Garden City Park, NY: Avery Publishing Group, 1996.

Graedon, J., et al., *The People's Pharmacy: Guide To Home And Herbal Remedies,* New York: St. Martin's Press, 1999.

Grøntved, A., et al., Ginger root against seasickness: a controlled trial on the open sea, *Acta Otolaryngol,* 105: 45–49, 1988.

Katiyar, S., et al., Inhibition of tumor promotion in SENCAR mouse skin by ethanol extract of *zingiber officinale* rhizome, *Cancer Res.,* 1;56: 1023–1030, 1996.

Langner, E., et al., Ginger: history and use, *Adv. Ther.,* 15: 25–44, 1998.

Lawless, J., *Aromatherapy And The Mind: The Psychological And Emotional Effects Of Essential Oils,* London: Thorsons, 1994.

Lipski, E., *Digestive Wellness,* Los Angeles: Keats Publishing, 2000.

Lumb, A.B., Effect of dried ginger on human platelet function, *Thromb. Haemost.,* 71(1): 110–111, 1994.

Micklefield, G.H., et al., Effects of ginger on gastroduodenal motility, *Int. J. Clin. Pharmacol. Ther.,* 37(7): 341–346, 1999.

Meyer, K., et al., *Zingiber officinale* (ginger) used to prevent 8-Mop associated nausea, *Dermatol. Nurs.,* 7: 242–244, 1991.

Morgan, J.P., The Jamaican ginger paralysis, *JAMA,* 248: 1864–1867, 1982.

Park, K., et al., Inhibitory effects of [6]-gingerol, a major pungent principle of ginger, on phorbol ester-induced inflammation, epidermal ornithine decarboxylase activity and skin tumor promotion in ICR mice, *Cancer Lett.,* 17;129(2): 139–44, 1998.

Rasoanaivo, P., et al., Essential oils of economic value in Madagascar: present state of knowledge, *HerbalGram,* 43: 31–39, 58–59, 1998.

Ryman, D., *Aromatherapy: The Encyclopedia Of Plants And Oils And How They Help You*, London: Judy Piatkus Publishers, Ltd., 1991.

Schulick, P., Ginger: common spice and wonder drug, Brattleboro, VT: Herbal Free Press, 1994.

Sreekumar, M.M., et al., Processing of fresh ginger: a technological breakthrough, *Indian Perfumer*, 43(3): 134–141, 1999.

Stewart, J., et al., Effects of ginger on motion sickness susceptibility and gastric function, *Pharmacology*, 42: 111–20, 1991.

Verma, S.K., et al., Effect of ginger on platelet aggregation in man, *Indian J. Med. Res.*, 98: 240–242, 1993.

Verma, S.K., et al., Ginger, fat and fibrinolysis, *Indian J. Med. Res.*, 55(2): 83–86, 2001.

Vimala, S., et al., Anti-tumor promoter activity in Malaysian ginger rhizobia used in traditional medicine, *Br. J. Cancer*, 80(1–2): 110–116, 1999.

Yoshikawa, M., et al., Stomachic principles in ginger. III. An anti-ulcer principle e. 6-gingesulfonic acid, and three monoacyldigalactosylglycerols, gingerglycolipids, A, B, and C, from *zingiberis Rhizoma* originating in Taiwan, *Chem. Pharm. Bull. (Tokyo)*, 42(6): 1226–1230, 1994.

Chapter 9

Earle, L., *Vital Oils*, London: Vermillion, 1994.

Gaydou, E.M., et al., Composition of the essential of ylang-ylang (*cananga odorata* hook fil. et Thomson forma genuine) from Madagascar, *Journal of Agriculture and Food Chemistry*, 34: 481, 1986.

Guibort, N.J.B.G., *Histoire Naturelle Des Drogues Simples, Ou Cours d'Histoire Naturelle*, Paris, France: J.B. Baillière & Fils, 1849.

Harding, J., *Secrets Of Aromatherapy*, East Sussex, England: Dorling Kindersley, 2000.

Keville, K., et al., *Aromatherapy: A Complete Guide To The Healing Art*, Santa Cruz, CA: The Crossing Press, 1995.

Kouwenhoven, A.P., *Madagascar: The Red Island*, Leiden, Holland: WINCO Publishing, 1995.

Lawless, J., *Aromatherapy And The Mind: The Psychological And Emotional Effects Of Essential Oils*, Wellingborough, England: Thorsons, 1994.

———, *The Complete Illustrated Guide To Aromatherapy*, Boston, MA: Element Books Ltd., 1997.

Marden, L., Madagascar: island at the end of the earth, *National Geographic*, 132;4: 443–487, October 1967.

Rasoanaivo, P., et al., Essential oils of economic value in Madagascar: present state of knowledge, *HerbalGram*, 43: 31–39, 58–59, 1998.

Rose, J., *The Aromatherapy Book*, Berkeley, CA: North Atlantic Books, 1992.

Chapter 10

Correll, D., Vanilla: its botany, history, cultivation and economic importance, *Econ. Bo.*, 7(4): 291–358, 1953.

DeVarigny, C., Fertilization of the vanilla flower by bees, *Bombay Nat. Hist.*, 4: 555–556, 1894.

Díaz, B., *The Discovery And Conquest Of Mexico*, New York: Farrar, Straus and Cudahy, 1956.

Gregory, L., et al., Parthenocarpic pod development by *vanilla planifolia* Andrews induced with growth-regulating chemicals, *Econ. Bot.*, 21: 351–357, 1967.

Hazen, J., *Vanilla*, San Francisco, CA: Chronicle Books, 1995.

Hillerman, F.E., et al., *An Introduction To The Cultivated Angraecoid Orchids Of Madagascar*, Portland, OR: Timber Press, 1986.

Hirsch, A., *Scentsational Sex: The Secret To Using Aroma For Arousal*, New York: Harper-Collins, 1998.

Marden, L., Madagascar: island at the end of the earth, *National Geographic*, 132:4: 443–487, October 1967.

Rain, P., *The Vanilla Cookbook*, Berkeley, CA: Celestial Arts, 1986.

Rasoanaivo, P., et al., Essential oils of economic value in Madagascar: present state of knowledge, *HerbalGram*, 43: 31–39, 58–59, 1998.

Reany, P., Curing chocolate cravings: people who wore skin patch ate fewer sweets, ABC News.com, http://abcnews.go.com/sections/living/DailyNews/chocaholic0724.html, 2000.

Stratton, A., *The Great Red Island*, New York: Charles Scribner's Sons, 1964.

Vanilla thriller, *Economist*, 363; 8269: 67, April 20, 2002.

Wood, D., Aromatherapy, *Magical Blend Magazine*, 60: 67–71, 1998.

Chapter 11

Arpaia, M.R., Effects of *centella asiatica* extract on mucopolysaccharide metabolism in subjects with varicose veins, *Int. J. Clin. Pharmacol. Res.*, 10(4): 229–233, 1990.

Boiteau, P., and Ratsimamanga, A.R., Asiaticoside extracted from *Centella asiatica*, its therapeutic uses in healing of experimental or refractory wounds, leprosy, skin tuberculosis, and lupus, *Therapie*, 11: 125–149, 1956.

Bosse, J.P., Clinical study of a new antikeloid agent, *Ann. Plast. Surg.*, 3(1): 13–21, 1979.

Chen, Y.J., et al., The effect of tetrandrine and extracts of *centella asiatica* on acute radiation dermatitis in rats, *Biol. Pharm. Bull.*, 22(7): 703–706, 1999.

Chopra, R.N., *Chopra's Indigenous Drugs Of India*, Calcutta, India: Dhur and Sons Ltd., 1958.

Freeman, R.G., et al., eds., *Clinical Dermatology*, New York: Harper & Row, 1976.

Guseva, N.G., Madécassol treatment of systemic and localized scleroderma, *Ter. Arkh.* 70(5): 58–61, 1998.

MacKay, D., Hemorrhoids and varicose veins: a review of treatment options, *Altern. Med. Rev.*, 6(2): 126–140, 2001.

Mallol, J., et al., Prophylaxis of *striae gravidarum* with a topical formulation: a double-blind trial, *Int. J. Cosmetic Sci.*, 13: 1–57, 1991.

Roche Nicholas Laboratories, Serdex Division, *Centella asiatica*, European Pharmacopoeia/Monograph 1498, 2001.

Sampson, J.H., et al., *In vitro* keratinocyte antiproliferant effect of *centella asiatica* extract and triterpenoid saponins, *Phytomedicine*, 8(3): 230–235, 2001.

Suguna, L., et al., Effects of *centella asiatica* extract on dermal wound healing in rats, *Indian. J. Exp. Biol.*, 34 (12): 1208–1211, 1996.

Sunikumar, P.S., et al., Evaluation of topical formulations of aqueous extract of *centella asiatica* on open wounds in rats, *Indian J. Exp. Biol.*, 36(6): 569–572, 1998.

Teuber, S.S., Saunders, R.L., Halpern, G.M., et al., Elevated serum silicon levels in women with silicone gel breast implants, *Biol. Trace. Elem. Res.*, 48: 121–130, 1995.

Chapter 12

Duke, J.A., *Handbook Of Medicinal Herbs*, Boca Raton, FL: CRC Press, 1985.

Freudenberger, K., Tree and land tenure: using rapid appraisal to study natural resource management: a case study from Anivorano, Madagascar, *Food*

And Agriculture Organization Of The United Nations, www.fao.org/forestry/FON/FONP/cfu/pub/en/cs/cs10/cs1000-e.stm, 1995.

Guichon, A., La superficie des formations forestières à Madagascar, *Revue Forestière Française,* 6: 408–411, 1960.

Jarosz, L., Defining and explaining tropical deforestation: shifting cultivation and population growth in colonial Madagascar (1896–1940), *Economic Geography,* 4: 366–380, 1993.

Jenkins, M.D., ed., *Madagascar: An Environmental Profile,* Cambridge, MA: IUCN, 1987.

Kouwenhoven, A.P., *Madagascar: The Red Island,* Leiden, Holland: WINCO Publishing, 1995.

Kull, C.A., Madagascar's burning issue, *Environment,* 44; 3: 8, April 2002.

Swerdlow, J.L., Nature's Rx, *National Georgraphic,* 197; 4: 98–117, April 2000.

Index

A

Acid reflux, 99
Acne, 2, 43, 62, 70
Acqua di Gio (Armani), 107
Adrenal glands, 70, 127
Aging, 86
Agni, 98
Agriculture. *See* Slash-and-burn agriculture; Sustainable agriculture.
AIDS, 90
Albius, Edmond, 116
Alcohol distillation, 37
Alexander the Great, 95
Alexandrian laurel. *See Calophyllum inophyllum.*
Allergies, 82, 89–90
American Dispensatory, 118
Analects, 95
Andrianampoinimerina, King, 23, 24
Anorexia, 97
Antaimoro tribe, 20, 21
Antananarivo, 23–24, 27
Antacids, 122
Antibacterial agents, 2, 86–88
Antifungal agents, 88–89, 90

Antilles vanilla. *See* Guadeloupe vanilla.
Antimicrobial agents, 2, 70–72, 82, 86–88
Antisiranana, 6, 26
Antitoxidants, 82, 85–86
Antongil Bay, 22
Anxiety, 62, 97, 122–123
Aphrodisiacs, 3, 97, 105, 108, 109, 111, 113, 114, 117–118, 124
Apicius, 95
Apple pie, 84
Aqua Admirabilis. *See* Eau de Cologne.
Aromacology Patch Company, 124
Aromathérapie, 38
Aromathérapie: traitement des maladies par les essences des plantes, 38
Aromatherapy, 2, 3–4, 29, 31, 32, 38–39, 70, 82, 97, 105, 108–109, 139, 140
Aromatherapy: The Encyclopedia of Plants and Oils and How They Help You, 98
Aromatherapy Quarterly, 31
Aromatic ravensare, 53, 54

Art of Aromatherapy, 38

Arthritis, 48, 98

Asarum canadense. See Wild ginger.

Asiatic acid, 127

Asiaticoside, 126, 127, 128, 130

Aspergillus, 89

Asthma, 126, 135

Augagneur, Victor, 135

Austronesians, 17–18

Avicenna, 37

Avozo oil. *See* Havozo oil.

Azoles, 90

Aztecs, 113

B

Babylon, 34

Bacteria, 2, 86–88

Bad breath, 86

Bamboo, 15

Bantus, 20

Bastard cinnamon. *See* Cassia.

Bauhin, Gaspard, 59

Beach calophyllum. *See*
    Calophyllum inophyllum.

Beagle (ship), 47

Beautiful (Estée Lauder), 107

Beauty leaf. *See Calophyllum
    inophyllum.*

Beefsteak plant, 88

Benzoic acid, 88

Benzoin gum, 88

Bergamot, 40

Beta-carotene, 86

Beta-sesquiphellandrene, 101

Betsimisaraka tribe, 117

Betsiboka River, 11

Bintangor tree, 49

Biodiversity, 10, 14–15, 50, 131

Birdwood, George, 70

Bisabolene, 93

Blavatsky, Helena Patrovna, 13

Blisters, 43

Blood circulation, 62, 82, 97, 126,
    127

Blood clots, 101, 102

Blood pressure, high. *See*
    Hypertension.

Blood sugar, 83

Boils, 2, 48, 62

*Book of a Thousand and One
    Nights*, 19

Book of Exodus (30:34), 36

*Book of Many Exotic Plants. See
    Exoticorum Libri Decem.*

Book of Mark (14:3–10), 35

Borman, Joannis, 60

Bourbon geraniums, 57–64
    medicinal uses, 62–63
    shopping for, 63–64
    See also Geraniums;
        Pelargoniums.

Bourbon vanilla, 111, 116, 121

Bowen, John, 22

Brahminoside, 126

Brahmoside, 126

Brain Research and Essential Oils,
    31

Bronchitis, 126

Burns, 2, 3, 43, 48, 62, 126

C

Calanolide A, 49

Calanolide B, 49

Calocoumarin-A, 50

Calophyllum inophyllum, 2, 43–50
    medicinal uses, 43, 48–50
    names, 45–46

non-medicinal uses, 44–45

safety, 45

spread, 46–48

Calaphyllum langerum. See Bintangor tree.

Camphor, 75

Camphor laurel. *See* Ravintsara.

Canadian snakeroot. *See* Wild ginger.

Canaga adoratum, 108

Canaga odorata. See Ylang-ylang.

Canaga oil, 108

Cancer, 67

    skin, 50, 103

    See also Leukemia, pediatric; Lymphoma, gastric.

Candida, 89

Candida albicans, 90

Candidiasis, 90

Canoes, 18, 46

Carbon dioxide extraction, 39

Cardamom, 86, 119

Carmelite water, 37

Carminatives, 82

Carnations, 59–60

Carrier oils, 30, 42, 43, 109

Cartilage, 126

Cassia, 75–77, 81

Catharanthus roseus. See Madagascar periwinkle.

Cattle, 20

Cayce, Edgar, 13

Cedarwood, 34

Cellulite, 3, 97, 126

Centella asiatica, 3, 125–130

    medicinal use, 127–130

    names, 125

Cerve, Wishar, 13

Ceylon. *See* Sri Lanka.

Ceylon cinnamon. *See* Cinnamon.

Chameleons, 15–16

Champs-Elysées (Guerlain), 107

Chanel No. 5, 107

Charaka Samhita, 98

Chemotypes, 40–41, 66–67

Chemovar. *See* Chemotype.

Chewing gum, 86

Chicken pox, 62

Chills, 70, 95

Chinese cassia. *See* Cassia.

Chinese cinnamon. *See* Cassia.

Chlorine, 71, 72

Chocolate, 81, 111, 113, 117–118, 124

Chocotatl, 113–114

Cicatritization, 48

Cineol, 52, 55, 66

Cinnamaldehyde, 75, 76, 77, 86–87, 89

Cinnamomum burmannii, 77

Cinnamomum camphora. See Ravintsara.

Cinnamomum loureirii, 77

Cinnamomum zeylanicum. See Cinnamon.

Cinnamon, 2, 29, 30, 34, 73–90

    cultivation, 74, 77–78, 81

    history, 78–81

    in the Bible, 78–79

    medicinal use, 81–90

    species, 75–77

Citronella, 137

Clove oil, 121

Cloves, 88

Clusius, Carolus, 114

Coca-Cola, 122

Cocoa butter, 46

Coconuts, 46

Coelacanth, 17
Cola drinks, 75
Cold sores, 43
Cold-press extraction, 39
Colds, 2, 51, 92, 95, 101
Collagen, 3, 126, 127, 128, 130
Collins, Catherine, 123–124
Columbus, Christopher, 96
Comoro Islands, 9
Complementary Therapy Nurse Midwifery, 83
Concentration, mental, 2, 70, 127
Confucius, 95
Conservation International, 131
Continental drift, 13
Coppices, 74
Cortés, Hernando, 113
Costa Rico, 136
Coughs, 70, 113
Coumadin, 49, 50
Coumarins, 49, 50, 76, 120–121
Cranberries, 88
Crave Control, 124
Crown charka, 127
CTCL. *See* Cutaneous T-cell lymphoma (CTCL).
Culpepper, Nicholas, 69
Cutaneous T-cell lymphoma (CTCL), 100

D

Darwin, Charles, 47
De Commerson, Philibert, 7, 9
De l'Écluse, Charles. *See* Clusius, Carolus.
De Re Coquinaria, 95
De Systema Naturae, 60–61
De Tournefort, Joseph Pitton, 68–69
Dental plaque, 86

Depression, 63, 70, 82, 108, 109, 122
Dermatitis, 2
Diabetes, 2, 82, 83–84, 135
Diamond, Jared, 18
Diarrhea, 81
Dias, Diogo, 21
Díaz, Bernal, 113
Diégo Suarez. *See* Antsiranana.
Digestion, 82, 95, 97, 99
Dilo oil. *See Calophyllum inophyllum*.
Dioscorides, 29, 36, 95
Discovery and Conquest of Mexico, 113
Distillation. *See* Alcohol distillation; Fractional distillation; Steam distillation.
Dizziness, 62
Drift seeds, 46
Du Barry, Comtesse, 118
Dutch East India Company, 61, 81

E

Ear aches, 70
Eau de Cologne, 37 93
Ecotourism, 11, 131, 136–137
Eczema, 43, 62, 127
8-methoxypsoralen. *See* 8-MOP.
8-MOP, 100
Eighth Continent, 21, 132
Eli Lilly Pharmaceuticals, 135
Elizabeth I, Queen, 96
Endemism, 7, 131
Endorphins, 32
Enfleurage, 39
English Physitian; or An Astrologo-physical Discourse of the Vulgar Herbs of the Nation, 69

Enkephalins, 32

Environmental fragrancing, 38

Epstein-Barr virus, 50, 102

Erectile dysfunction. *See* Sexual dysfunction.

Erzulie, 68

Escape (Calvin Klein), 107

Essential oils, 1, 2, 3-4, 8, 9-10, 11, 29-30, 34-36, 38, 39-42, 137-138, 139, 140
   extraction methods, 39-40
   safety, 42
   shopping for, 41-42, 141-142

Esters, 108

Estragole. *See* Methyl-chavicol.

Eugenol, 66, 75, 76, 77

European Commission on Health and Human Protection, 67

Every, Henry, 22

Exotic sweet basil oil, 65
   safety, 67

Exoticorum Libri Decem, 114

F

Fagot cassia. *See Cinnamomum burmannii.*

Fateh Mohammed (ship), 22

Febrifuge, 122

Fibroblasts, 63, 127, 128

Fischer-Rizzi, Susanne, 32

Flightless aepyornis, 16, 19

Foraha oil. *See Calophyllum inophyllum.*

Fort Dauphin. *See* Taolañaro.

Fractional distillation, 108

Franco-Hova Wars, 25, 26, 27

Frankincense, 33, 34, 36

Free radicals, 85-86

French vanilla, 122

Frigidity. *See* Sexual dysfunction.

Fungi, 2, 82

G

Galanolactone, 99

Galbanum, 34

Galen, 95

Galliéni, Joseph-Simon, 9

Gardner's Dictionary, 114

Gas-liquid chromatography, 41

Gastritis, 85

Gattefossé, René-Maurice, 38

Geraniums, 59-61, 137
   See also Bourbon geraniums; Pelargoniums.

Geranoil, 93

Gerard, John, 62, 70

Ginger, 2, 29, 91-105, 137, 138
   cultivation, 93-95
   history, 95-97
   medicinal use, 97-103

Ginger ale, 97, 98, 99

Ginger beer, 96

Ginger Jake paralysis. *See* Jake leg.

Gingerbread, 96

Gingeroles, 93

Ging-i-Saway (ship), 22

Glucose. *See* Blood sugar.

Glutathione (GSH), 86

Golden Age of Piracy, 22-23

Gondwanaland, 14

Gout, 69

Great Herbal. See Pen Tsao Ching.

Greek Orthodox Church, 68

GSH. *See* Glutathione (GSH).

Guadelouupe vanilla, 122

Gum benjamin. *See* Benzoin gum.

Gunn, C., 47

H

H. pylori. See Helicobacter pylori.

Haeckel, Ernst Heinrich, 12–13

Hair, 70, 106, 109

Havozo. See Ravensara aromatica.

Havozo oil, 53

Hazomanitra. See Ravensara aromatica.

Head lice, 81, 82–83

Headaches, 51, 109

Healing Trail, 139–140

Heart attacks, 101–102

Heartburn, 99

Helicobacter pylori, 82, 85, 99

Heliotropin, 123

Hemorrhoids, 62, 129, 130

Henry VIII, King, 96

Herbs, pungent, 98

Herball or Generall Historie of Plants, 62, 70

Hernandez, Francisco, 114

Herodotus, 79

Hirsch, Alan, 124

Histoplasma capsulatum, 89

HIV, 2, 43, 49

Ho wood oil, 53, 54–55

Hodgkin's disease, 131, 135, 136

Holy basil, 67–68, 70

Hornac, J., 134

Hot flashes, 63

Hypertension, 3, 62, 109, 135

Hypochlorhydria, 85

Hyssop, 32

I

I am Ramtha, 13

IgE, 89

Immune system, 127

Impotence. See Sexual dysfunction.

Indian ginger. See Wild ginger.

Indian laurel. See Calophyllum inophyllum.

Indigénat, 27

Indonesian cinnamon. See Cinnamomum burmannii.

Inflammation, joint, 98

Infrared spectrometry, 41

Insect bites, 43, 106, 127

Insect repellants, 63, 70, 122

Insomnia, 70, 109

Institutiones Rei Herbariæ, 68–69

Insulin, 82, 83

International Wildlife Federation, 136

Isabella, Queen, 96

Itching, 127

Ivoloina Botanical Park, 9

J

Jake, 96–97

Jake leg, 96

Jardin des Pamplemousses, 9, 81

Jarosz, Lucy, 135

Jasmine, 30, 39

Java cassia. See Cinnamomum burmannii.

Jefferson, Thomas, 62, 114–115

Jejolava, 20

Jesus, 35

John Bartram Botanical Gardens, 62

Johnson, John, 62

Judas Iscariot, 35

K

Kananga. See Ylang-ylang.

Keloids. See Scar tissue.

Kidd, William, 22
Kilopilopitsofy, 16
Kily, 136
King, John, 118
Knight, J. Z., 13
Krishna, Lord. *See* Vishnu.

L

L'Heritier, Charles-Louis, 60
La Buse, Oliver, 22
Lambert, Joseph-François, 25, 26
Lambert Charter, 25, 26
Laterite, 11
Laurasia, 14
Lavaka, 10
Lavender, 38, 124
Lemongrass, 40, 109, 137
Lemur 2000 Inc.-Phael-Flor USA,
    141–142
Lemur Tours, 139, 140
Lemuria, 12–13, 14
*Lemuria: The Lost Continent of the
    Pacific,* 13
Lemurs, 16
    giant, 15
Leprosy, 43, 48, 95, 126, 127
Leukemia, pediatric, 131, 135, 136
Lignin, 121
Limbic system, 32
Limonene, 93
Linalool, 55, 66, 108
Linnaeus, Carl, 59–61
Lipase, 93
Lipid peroxidation, 86
Logging, 134
Longevity, 127
Lost Lemuria, 13
Louis XV, King, 118

Lymphoma, gastric, 85

M

Macassar oil, 106–106
Madagascar periwinkle, 15, 131,
    135–136
Madagascar, 1–2, 4, 6, 7–28,
    131–132, 139, 140
  British in, 24
  Christianity, 24, 25, 26
  climate, 10
  economy, 8, 9, 27–28, 134–135
  environment, 8–9
  fauna, 11, 15–16
  fires, 131–132
  flora, 11, 14–15
  French colonial rule, 27
  French in, 24, 25, 26
  geography, 7, 8, 10
  history, 17–28
  horticulture, 9
  independence, 27–28, 134–135
  Islam, 21
  language, 19, 20
  map, 5
  megafauna, 16–17
  place names, 4, 19, 20
  population, 11
  tribes, 18–19, 21–22, 23
  traveling to, 143–146
Madecassic acid, 126, 127
Madécassol, 128, 129, 130
Madecassoside, 126, 127, 128
Madeleines, 31
Magnetic resonance imaging (MRI),
    122–123
Malagasies, 6
Malaria, 136

Manne, Sharon, 122–123
Marie-Suzanne, Sister, 48
Marotaina, 74
Marshall, Barry, 85
Mary Magdalene, 35
Massage oils, 2, 33, 38, 52, 70
Mauritius, 9, 24
Maury, Marguerite, 38
Mayeur, Nicolas, 23
McLaughlin, John, 97
Measles, 136
MediChem Research, 49
Megaleion, 78
Melipona bee, 115
Menopause, 109
Menstruation, 70, 97, 135
   cramps, 69, 82
   disorders, 63
Merino tribe, 18, 19, 23–27
Methyl-chavicol, 66, 67
Methyl-cinnamate, 66
Methylhydroxychalcone (MHCP), 84
Mexico, 112–114, 115, 117
MHCP. See Methylhydroxychalcone
   (MHCP).
Michaux, André, 9
Microbes, 2, 70–72, 88
Mid-Atlantic Ridge, 14
Miller, Philip, 114
Miscarriages, 70, 97
Mohammed, 95
Mononucleosis, 2, 102
Montezuma, King, 113
Morgan, Hugh, 114
Morren, Charles, 115, 116
Motion sickness, 2, 98–99, 100
Mount Maromokotro, 10
Mouthwash, 86

Muddling Through in Madagascar,
   143
Murphy, Dervla, 143
Muscles, aching, 70
Musk, 40
Myrrh, 34, 36, 82

N

Napoléon III, Emperor, 25
Nard oil. *See* Spikenard.
National Academy of Science, 86
National Cancer Institute, 49
Nausea, 2, 97, 99, 100–101, 109, 122
Neral, 93
Nero, 78
Neuritis, 48
Nipagin A, 88
Nostra Senhora (ship), 22
Nosy Bé, 105, 106
Nosy Boraha, 6, 22, 23
Nosy Manitra. *See* Nosy Bé.

O

Ocimum basilicum. See Sweet basil.
Oleoresin, 91
Ombiasy, 20, 21, 126, 136
On Experiences, 118
Orange oil, 82, 109
Orchids, 15, 111–112
Oxidation, 86

P

Padang cinnamon. *See*
   Cinnamomum burmannii.
Palms, 15
Pancreas, 93
Pangaea, 13
Patchouli, 40, 109

Pediculicides, 83

Pediculus capitis. See Head lice.

Pelargonium roseum. See Bourbon geraniums.

Pelargoniums, 2, 40, 57–64

Pen Tsao Ching, 95

Pennywort. *See Centella asiatica.*

Perfumes, 33–38, 91, 105, 106, 107, 111, 118

    classification, 40

    in the Bible, 34–36, 78–79

Phael-Flor, 51, 77–78, 131, 137–138

Phlebitis, 126

Photopheresis, 100

Piesse, Charles, 40

Pirates, 22–23

Plague, 96

Plate tectonics, 13–14

Pliny the Elder, 29, 36, 79–80

Plums, 88

Poison (Christian Dior), 107

Poisoning, 95

    shellfish, 97

Poivre, Pierre, 9, 81

Polo, Marco, 19, 80, 96

Pomades, 106

Poppaea, 78

Poucher, William, 40

Practice of Aromatherapy. See Aromathérapie: traitement des maladies par les essences des plantes.

Pregnancy, 70, 97, 130

Premenstrual syndrome, 63, 109

Primates, 16

Princess of Tai, 95

Prohibition, 96

Protease, 93

Proust, Marcel, 31

Proverbs 7 (16–18), 78–79

Psalms 45 (7–8), 35–36

Psoriasis, 43, 128–129

Puranas, 68

Pygmy hippo, 16

Q

Qi, 97

Quarterly Journal of Science, 12

R

Radama I, King, 23

Radama II, King, 25, 26

Rain, Patricia, 121

Rainforests, 1, 8, 11, 15, 131, 133, 134, 136

Rainilaiarivory, 26, 27

Rainivoninahitriniony, 26

Rajasinha II, King, 80

Rakotomalala, Roger, 139, 140

Ramboatiana, Rolland, 136, 138

Ramtha, 13

Ranavalona I, Queen, 24–25

Ranavalona II, Queen, 26

Ranavalona III, Queen, 26

Ranavalona the Cruel. *See* Ranavalona I, Queen.

Rasoaherina, Queen, 26

Ratsimamanga, Rakoto, 126

Ratsiraka, Didier, 28

Ravalomanana, Marc, 28

Ravenala (Musaceae), 12

Ravensara aromatica, 2, 53–54

Ravensare. *See Ravensara aromatica.*

Ravintsara, 2, 51–55, 137

    classification, 52–53

    medicinal uses, 51

Remembrance of Things Past, 31

Rerum Medicarum Novae Hispaniae Thesaurus, 114

Respiratory tract mycosis, 88–89

Réunion, 9, 24, 58, 105, 115

Réunion basil oil. *See* Exotic sweet basil oil.

Rheumatism, 52, 69, 70, 136

Rhinovirus B, 101

Rhinoviruses, 101

Rhizomes, 92–93

Rice, 18, 23, 134–135

Romazava, 96

Rootstock. *See* Rhizomes.

Rose geraniums. *See* Bourbon geraniums.

Rose, Jeanne, 81, 109

Rose water, 37

Roses, 40

Rosy periwinkle. *See* Madagascar periwinkle.

Rova, 74

Rowland's Macassar oil. *See* Macassar oil.

Ryman, Daniele, 98

S

Saffron, 119

Saigon cinnamon. *See Cinnamomum loureirii.*

Sampy, 25, 26

Sandalwood, 109

Sarawak, 49–50

Sàvoka, 10

Scabies, 81

Scar tissue, 126, 127
   hypertrophic, 130

Scent, 3–4, 29, 32
   psychology of, 30–33

Sciatica, 48

Sclater, Philip Lutley, 12

Scleroderma, 129

Scopolamine, 100

Scorpio, 68

Scorpions, 68

Scott-Elliot, William, 13

Seeds, 46–48

Secret Doctrine, 13

Secret of Life and Youth, 38

Serotonin, 32, 123–124

Sesquiterpenes, 108, 138

Sexual dysfunction, 97, 109, 118, 124

Sézary syndrome, 100

Shen Nung, 95

Shingles, 48

Shogaol, 98

Sick building syndrome, 38

Siegesbeck, Johann, 61

Siegesbeckia orientalis, 61

Skin, 2, 43, 63, 97, 126
   ailments, 43, 48, 62, 70
   dry, 2, 62, 109
   test, 42
   See also Wounds; Wrinkles.

Slash-and-burn agriculture, 131, 132–133

Slave trade, 20, 23, 24, 116

Smell. *See* Scent.

Snake bites, 70, 106

Socrates, 33–34

Solvent extraction, 39

Song of Solomon (4:13–15), 34

Sonnerat, Pierre, 9

Sore throats, 81

"Sowing basil," 68

Species Plantarum, 59

Spice trade, 21, 34, 79–81, 95

Spices, 33, 96

Spider veins, 129

Spikenard, 34, 35

Spiny Desert, 10–11

Sri Lanka, 80–81

Sri Lankan cinnamon. *See* Cinnamon.

St. Mary's Island. *See* Nosy Boraha.

Steam distillation, 39

Steele, John, 31

Stomach ailments, 51, 99, 113, 122

Stress, 2, 63, 70, 109

Stretch marks, 130

Striae. *See* Stretch marks.

Sunburn, 43

Sunscreens, 63

Sustainable agriculture, 77, 137

Svoboda, Gordon, 135

Sweet basil, 2, 29, 40, 65–72, 137
  folklore, 67–69
  medicinal use, 69–70
  non-medicinal use, 70–72
  See also Exotic sweet basil oil; True sweet basil oil.

Syphilis, 126

T

T cells, 100, 128

Tahiti, 45

Tahitian vanilla, 111, 121–122

Tamanu oil. *See* Calophyllum inophyllum.

Taolañaro, 4, 21–22

Tavy, 134

Taylor, John, 22

Temple of Solomon, 32

Tenrecs, 16

Tew, Thomas, 22

Therapie, 126

Thomas, Henry, 23

Thoth, 33

Thrush, 90

Tiger's grass. *See Centella asiatica.*

Tikis, 45

Tisserand, Robert, 38

Toilet-water, 37

Tom's of Maine, 91

Tonka bean, 129

Tooth paste, 86, 91

Totonaca, 113

Totonocopan, 112–113

Tradescant, John, 62

Triorthocresylphosphate (TOCP), 96

Triterpenoid compounds, 125, 127

True sweet basil oil, 65

Tsaratanana Massif, 15

Tuberculosis, 127

Tulsi Vivaha, 68

Tyson, Peter, 21, 132

U

U.S. Agency for International Development (USAID), 78, 136

U.S. Food and Drug Administration, 67

U.S. Food, Drug and Cosmetic Act of 1938, 76

U.S. Library of Congress. Jefferson Papers collection, 115

Ulcers, 48
  chronic duodenal, 85
  skin, 126
  stomach, 2, 82, 85, 99

Ultraviolet (UV) light, 103

Unguents, 33, 34

University of Illinois at Chicago, 49
Urease, 85

V

Valiha, 20
Valley Fever, 88
Valnet, Jean, 38
Vanilla, 3, 111–124
    cultivation, 119
    curing, 119–120
    extract, 120–121
    history, 112–117
    medicinal uses, 122–124
    pollination, 115–116, 119
    rustling, 119
Vanilla Cookbook, 121
Vanilla planifolia. See Boubon
    vanilla.
Vanilla pompona. See Guadeloupe
    vanilla.
Vanilla tahitensis. See Tahitian
    vanilla.
Vanillin, 120
Vanmilla fragrans. See Bourbon
    vanilla.
Varicose veins, 3, 62, 97, 126, 129,
    130
Vazimba, 17
Veins. *See* Spider veins; Varicose
    veins.
Vetiver, 137
Vietnamese cinnamon. *See*
    Cinnamomum loureirii
Vinblastine, 135, 136
Vincristine, 135, 136
Vintana, 21

Vishnu, 67–68
Vitamin C, 86
Vitamin E, 86
Vitamin K, 49
Voafotsy, 136
Voodoo, 68

W

Warfarin, 49
Warren, Robin, 85
Wegener, Alfred, 13–14
Weight control, 123
White Pigeon (ship), 22
Wild ginger, 92
Willoughby, Digby, 26
World Wildlife Fund, 131, 136
Wounds, 2, 48, 98, 126, 127, 128
Wrinkles, 2, 127

X

Xanat, Princess, 113

Y

Yardley's Brown Windsor soaps, 75
Yeasts, 2, 83, 88
Ylang-ylang, 3, 30, 82, 105–109
    cultivation, 107–108
    grading, 108

Z

Zebus, 20
Zimmermann, Bezar, 118
Zingerone, 93
Zingiber officinale. See Ginger.
Zingiberene, 93